THE VETERINARIANS' GUIDE TO
NATURAL REMEDIES FOR CATS

THE VETERINARIANS' GUIDE TO
NATURAL REMEDIES
FOR
CATS

**Safe and Effective Alternative Treatments and Healing
Techniques from the Nation's Top Holistic Veterinarians**

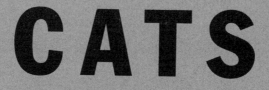

MARTIN ZUCKER

**Foreword by Carvel Tiekert, DVM
Founder, American Holistic Veterinary Medical Association**

Three Rivers Press • *New York*

Note to the Reader

This book about natural remedies is intended for educational purposes and is not meant to replace veterinary medical care or any therapeutic program recommended by a veterinarian.

If your cat has a health problem, see a qualified veterinarian, preferably one who integrates holistic methods and natural remedies in his or her practice.

The recommendations contained in this book involve practices and remedies based on the experiences of individual veterinarians. Such recommendations are of a general nature and may not apply to your particular animal's condition.

Neither the author nor the publisher can be held responsible for any adverse reactions to the recipes, recommendations, or ideas in this book.

Copyright © 1999 by Martin Zucker
All rights reserved. No part of this book may be reproduced or transmitted in any form or by any means, electronic or mechanical, including photocopying, recording, or by any information storage and retrieval system, without permission in writing from the publisher.

Published by Three Rivers Press 201 East 50th Street, New York, New York 10022. Member of the Crown Publishing Group.

Random House, Inc. New York, Toronto, London, Sydney, Auckland
www.randomhouse.com

THREE RIVERS PRESS is a registered trademark of Random House, Inc.

Printed in the United States of America

Design by Cynthia Dunne

Library of Congress Cataloging-in-Publication Data
Zucker, Martin.
    The veterinarians' guide to natural remedies for cats: safe and effective alternative treatments and healing techniques from the nation's top holistic veterinarians / by Martin Zucker; foreword by Carvel Tiekert.—1st pbk. ed.
    Includes bibliographical references.
    1. Cats—Diseases—Alternative treatment.   2. Cats—Health.
3. Holistic veterinary medicine.   I. Title.
SF985.Z83 1999
636.8'089—dc21   99–23724
                                                                                      CIP

ISBN 0–609–80373–5

10 9 8 7 6 5 4 3 2 1

First Edition

To Carole and Chantale with a heart full of love.

Acknowledgments

I AM DEEPLY grateful to the many veterinarians who generously shared their vast and precious healing knowledge. Among them are true pioneers whose visions and methods are being widely applied today as more and more veterinarians realize that good medicine is not limited just to surgery and drugs, but is also about feeding quality food and using remedies that work the best and are the least invasive and the least toxic. Thanks to Nino Aloro, DVM; Wendell O. Belfield, DVM; Jan Bellows, DVM; Karen Bentley, DVM; Carolyn S. Blakey, DVM; Ron Carsten, DVM; Christina Chambreau, DVM; Roger DeHaan, DVM; Joseph Demers, DVM; Edmund R. Dorosz, DVM; Lynne M. Friday, DVM; Maria Glinski, DVM; Robert Goldstein, VMD; Stan Gorlitsky, DVM; Mark Haverkos, DVM; Shannon Hines, DVM; A. Greig Howie, DVM; Jody Kincaid, DVM; Charles Loops, DVM; Paul McCutcheon, DVM; Donna Starita Mehan, DVM; Alfred J. Plechner, DVM; William Pollak, DVM; Pedro Luis Rivera, DVM; Allen Schoen, DVM; Nancy Scanlan, DVM; Tejinder Sodhi, DVM; Carvel Tiekert, DVM; Thomas E. Van Cise, DVM; Pamela Wood-Krzeminski, DVM; Susan G. Wynn, DVM; Michele Yasson DVM; and Jean Hofve, DVM, for not only sharing her special cat knowledge, but also for reviewing the manuscript, diagnosing the flaws, and making winning suggestions.

I am particularly proud to have the voice of Norman Ralston, DVM, in this book. Ralston, a great holistic pioneer of veterinary medicine for more than fifty years, passed away in 1999. The holistic community will miss him very much.

Special thanks to PJ Dempsey, senior editor at Crown Publishing Group, whose friendship and sure handling of the editorial reins steered this book across the finish line. And to Bob Silverstein, of Quicksilver Books, a superb agent and caring friend.

Contents

Foreword

THIS BOOK IS filled with practical ideas and recommendations. If you use the information appropriately, you can create optimally healthy cats functioning at the very highest level of vitality that their genetic programming allows.

To do so, to achieve this desirable goal, you need to become an educated caregiver for your companion animal. Your role is critical. Above all, you must really get to know your cat. You need to become so familiar with your animal when it is healthy that you can recognize the first signs of illness right away and take remedial action promptly.

By knowing your animal, you need to regard it from a caregiver's perspective. Look at its ears, at its teeth. Look between the toes. Look underneath. Anything that is abnormal is judged in the relationship to what is regarded as normal. And what may be normal for one animal may not be normal for another. Knowing your cat intimately brings you in closer contact and improves your mutual bonding, making the experience of being guardian that much richer.

By knowing your animal, you can also help us—the veterinarians—do our job as partners in helping your animal to better health. Just as you (and not somebody with an M.D. after his or her name) are ultimately responsible for your own health, so you are also ultimately responsible for the health of your cat. My role as veterinarian is as consultant and facilitator. I can make all the recommendations in the world, but if you don't do the work at home and make it a team effort—both to try the recommendations and to report responses accurately—in many cases there won't be a proper resolution. You have to be involved.

You don't become healthy simply by taking a pill to get rid of a symptom or by undergoing an operation to eliminate something nasty in the body. These things don't create health. What counts the most is what you do over your lifetime—and the lifetime of your pet. Your actions create either chronic illness or chronic health. Unfortunately there are no magic bullets.

Most of the time, Western medicine is very good at handling acute care. It is also useful for diagnosis, and sometimes prognosis, and evaluating response to therapy. However, it doesn't have a good record for chronic disease. The problem is that the system is oriented to the elimination of symptoms. In many cases the symptom is the body's best response to a negative stimulus—for example, if you have pain in a joint due to arthritis, the body is telling you to take it easy. A conventional drug may make the pain go away, but the problem (inflammation) is still there, and you haven't helped the problem. Instead you may have aggravated it.

By comparison, when you use most natural therapies, if the pain goes away, it's because you have altered the course of the disease, *and the body no longer needs the symptom*.

This book is unique. It contains recommendations and ideas based on the clinical experience of many veterinarians who routinely use natural therapies and who know what works and what doesn't work. Health writer Marty Zucker has done us all an important service by gathering this wealth of professional experience and shaping it into a practical book for cat owners. His concept is to give you different options so that if one particular approach for condition "X" doesn't work, a second or third one might. Each cat, just as each person, is a different creature, with a unique set of individual needs, individual biochemistry, and individual reactions. It is important to remember that. So if one option that you read about and try doesn't work, go to another one. Zucker gives you options that veterinarians have used in their own practices with good results. Given the individuality of all creatures, human or animal, this is a very practical idea. One remedy might work for your cat but not for your neighbor's cat.

As you use this book keep one thing in mind. If you are dealing with what appears to be a minor problem, and your cat doesn't respond after you follow the advice you read here, don't wait until it's too late and your cat is nearly dead before you see your veterinarian. Besides the fact that it could cost you a lot more money, there may be nothing that can be done at that point.

As I said earlier, know your animal. That will help you as you consider the remedies and concepts in this book or, for that matter, any therapy your veterinarian recommends. I can't emphasize this point enough. You need to be able to evaluate progress or lack of it. You do that by knowing your animal.

Good luck in your search for optimum wellness for you and your pet.

Carvel Tiekert, DVM, Bel Air, Maryland
Founder, American Holistic Veterinary Medical Association

Introduction

"WHAT FOOD SHOULD I feed my cat?"

"What vitamins should I give my cat?"

"How do I give homeopathic medicines to my cat?"

"Is there a natural remedy I can use for my cat's constant scratching?"

Over the years many pet owners have asked me these types of questions because I am a health writer who has coauthored three previous books with veterinarians. The questions were posed by people looking for information on how to help their animals holistically. Most of them were unsure about how to start a natural healing program for their pets and were unable to get guidance from their veterinarians. Often they were concerned about veterinary prescriptions causing side effects and wanted to know how they could avoid medications. I am not a veterinarian, so I could speak only in general terms and share what I have learned from holistic veterinarians. Most of the time I would recommend that they consult with a holistic practitioner.

The repeated questions sparked an idea for a book that would provide pet owners with a practical introduction to the wide and wondrous world of natural healing. The idea matured into a plan to interview the leading veterinary experts and transform their clinical experience into books for dog and cat caregivers. In the process of bringing the plan to completion, I interviewed three dozen veterinarians with a combined experience of nine hundred years in practice—an average of about twenty-five years each. This book, and the accompanying book for dogs, are the final product: precious collections, I sincerely believe, of healing knowledge that can raise the health of pets to the highest possible level.

In this book you will find the following information:

- Dozens of natural remedies for common conditions of cats, with precise guidelines on how and when to use them and even how to get the fussiest of cats to take them.

- An informal, yet alarming, survey revealing widespread poor health among our feline population.
- Advice from nutritionally oriented veterinarians on how to improve your cat's diet. This is critical information. You cannot build a house on quicksand, and you can't build a healthy body with poor nutrition. Much of what is mass-merchandised to you as good, easy-to-serve pet food is really making your cat sick. Pet food manufacturers want you to believe their products are wholesome, but veterinarians believe otherwise.
- Quality pet food brands recommended by veterinarians.
- The supreme importance of feeding meat to cats.
- The "HIT list"—foods "high in trouble" and most likely to cause allergic reactions in cats.
- Recipes for weight loss. Obesity is not just a human problem. There is a major fat cat problem.
- Why you should brush your cat's teeth regularly.
- How to energize older cats and keep younger ones healthy.
- The real dangers of overvaccination and how you can prevent vaccine-related health problems.
- How to recognize stress—the frequent cause of behavioral or health problems in cats—and take practical steps to alleviate fear, anxiety, and other stressful emotions.
- Revelations about health-robbing hormonal-immune defects in many purebred cats, and increasingly in mixed breeds as well, that stem from questionable breeding practices. You will learn how to protect your animals from the suffering these defects cause.

Even though the recommendations throughout this book have been made by veterinarians, such general advice can never substitute for a firsthand examination, diagnosis, and treatment offered by an experienced professional. The book does not replace professional veterinary care. If your cat is being treated by a veterinarian, please share the information about any remedy or recommendation in the book that you wish to utilize. Many of the recommendations contained here have the ability to enhance and support ongoing treatments.

If your cat is in an obvious crisis, or if a problem persists, or if

symptoms appear to worsen after you begin using one of the recommended remedies, do not delay in consulting with a veterinarian.
If you are interested in the services of a holistic veterinarian, contact
the American Holistic Veterinary Medical Association in Bel Air,
Maryland, at 410-569-0795, and ask for the name of a nearby practitioner.

How to Use This Book

ALTERNATIVE MEDICINE ENCOURAGES you to take an active role in the health of your cat. Part 1 tells you why this is so necessary. As revealed in chapter 2, veterinarians are disturbed by a rise of serious illnesses among our companion animals. You must get involved to protect your pet.

The first commandment of better health is to feed your cat a better diet. Much of the pet food sold in the marketplace is loaded with inferior, highly processed ingredients lacking freshness and wholesomeness. Such food is blamed by veterinarians as a major cause of health problems. Chapter 3 tells you the startling facts about the quality of pet food that you will never learn from advertising claims. Chapter 4 shows you how to move up to a better diet and informs you why feeding meat to a cat is the most natural and probably the most beneficial single thing you can do for your animal. Here you will also find a checklist for recognizing whether your cat is eating a healthy—or not so healthy—diet. Chapter 5 is all about healthy add-ons to a base of quality commercial food. Chapter 6 gives you recipes for 100 percent home-prepared meals. Either way, you will be surprised at how little time you need in order to upgrade your cat to superior nutrition.

Part 1 also acquaints you with some of the major holistic approaches available to pet owners—such as acupuncture and homeopathy—and basics on vitamins, herbs, homeopathy, and flower essences. Some of the veterinarians have also shared wonderful healing massages—described in chapter 13—that you can easily administer to your cat.

Chapter 14 covers the controversial issue of vaccinations. Holistic veterinarians contend that pets are given too many vaccinations, a practice that often causes serious health problems. This chapter will include recommendations on how to prevent or minimize such problems.

What if nothing you read in this book, or any other book, or anything your veterinarian tries, helps a suffering cat? Many pets are genetically flawed because of horrendous breeding practices—so flawed, in fact, that they succumb to sickness early in life. In chapter 15 you will find information about two important tests that offer vital clues—and hope—for dealing with resistant, heartbreak cases.

In part 2, the main section of the book, you will find the natural remedies for many common conditions affecting cats. Conditions are listed *alphabetically*. For each condition, you will find individual recommendations grouped under the following categories: flower essences, herbs, homeopathic remedies, nutritional supplements, multiple approaches, and food and special diets.

As a consumer you are exposed to many advertising claims. The broadside of information can be confusing. When I set out to write this book my goal was to help steer pet owners to effective natural remedies. I asked each of the veterinarians I interviewed: "What are the remedies you use that work well repeatedly?" You will find their answers in part 2. Each recommendation that appears is listed with the name of the veterinarian who has used it successfully in practice. Some recommendations are simple, based on one remedy. Others involve giving multiple remedies.

Imagine a menu in a restaurant created by not just a single great chef, but by dozens of culinary masters. This book is like a "health menu of masters," filled with the health-building recipes from veterinarians who have been perfecting natural healing methods for many years. Their insights give you safe and powerful options to pick from—as a menu—for preventing common conditions, enhancing the healing process, and improving health. It is not possible to say which one of the several or more remedies listed under any given condition is the most effective. Each remedy or approach, however, has been used successfully by a veterinarian. Choose the option that fits your situation best. Keep in mind that each animal is an individual and may not respond to one particular remedy. That is why I included a variety of options for each condition. If one doesn't help, try another. Recommendations include product names, where to obtain the products, and specific instructions for dosages.

Part 2 begins with *general guidelines on dosages and administering remedies. Please read this section before looking up specific conditions.* Cats are quite the challenge when it comes to giving medicines, supplements, or remedies of any sort. Learn how the experts do it. There is information here for dosing fussy cats. Please read it. Natural remedies will never work unless you can get them into your cat. The advice here will make it easier on you...and your cat...and help you in your effort to protect and optimize the health of your pet.

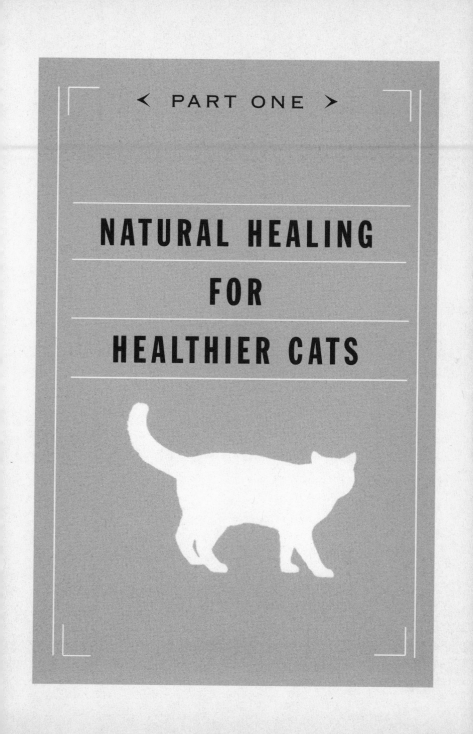

< PART ONE >

NATURAL HEALING

FOR

HEALTHIER CATS

Why Alternative Veterinary Medicine?

When you hear a veterinarian say, "We can't cure it," or, "All we can do is to try to control it," that's a good time to take the alternative approach if you haven't already done so.

—*Nancy Scanlan, DVM, Sherman Oaks, California*

THE ALTERNATIVE APPROACH? Alternative to what?

Simply put, it's an approach that bypasses the Western medical obsession with disease and symptoms and instead focuses on health and healing. It is an approach drawing millions of converts to holistic healers not only for themselves, but for their animals as well. It is a needed approach whose time has come.

Researchers say that as much as 40 percent of the population suffers from chronic ailments. Although our modern medical system has made astounding advances in emergency medicine, acute care treatment, and sophisticated diagnostics, the same system fails to effectively prevent or heal chronic disease. The system, in fact, promotes treatments, procedures, and drugs that often cause substantial—even deadly—adverse reactions and new symptoms.

Veterinarians describe a somewhat parallel situation in their field, an epidemic of chronic disease in which animals become sick and die well before their time. Modern veterinary medicine has also made remarkable progress in diagnostics, surgical treatments, and acute care, yet the profession's overall ability to deal with chronic disease leaves much to be desired. Conventional methods frequently relieve symptoms temporarily but fall short of healing animals or effectively raising their levels of health.

The typical style of medical practice is based largely on a pharmosurgical education taught at medical schools. But in recent years increasing numbers of both physicians and veterinarians have found a need to expand their horizons to other types of therapies—typically not taught in medical schools. These methods are categorized popularly as "alternative" or "holistic" practices.

Asked why they turned to holistic medicine, the veterinarians interviewed for this book gave similar answers:

- "The methods we were taught were too limiting."
- "I wasn't healing animals, only relieving their symptoms for a while."
- "I was dissatisfied with my ability to help my patients."
- "I was frustrated."

These veterinarians repeatedly told me they became increasingly aware of their failure to effectively stop the advance of chronic diseases that continued to destroy tissue and life force at deeper and deeper levels despite their treatments. And this is why, they said, they looked beyond, to other options, and became attracted to acupuncture, chiropractic, homeopathy, nutritional therapies using food, supplements, and herbs, and other natural healing traditions. Sometimes they used these newly learned methods alone, other times they practiced these methods in conjunction with drugs or surgery, dramatically improving the outcome of treatments. With these practices they found the means to turn around sick patients, optimize their health, and often extend life.

GENTLER OPTIONS THAT RALLY THE WHOLE BODY

Alternative practitioners say their methods harness and rally all the resources of the mind, body, and spirit—the whole person, the whole animal—and support the healing process rather than interfering with it. These methods revolve around a central concept as old as the art of healing itself: that each person, each living thing, possesses on a deep level the will and intelligence to be healthy and that these elements can and should be enlisted in effecting a cure.

The use of alternatives has caught on big time and today is revolutionizing the business and practice of Western medicine—both human and veterinary medicine. As *Time* magazine noted in a 1997 article, "Alternative medicine for pets may not be as widespread or well publicized as the human variety, but it's growing faster than a sprig of St. John's wort."

"Pet owners have recognized a bigger range of possibilities," says Thomas Van Cise, DVM, of Norco, California. "Alternative methods provide a gentler option when mainstream treatments, like surgery or powerful drugs, might be too extreme or cause too many adverse side effects. You can also treat and heal many cases naturally for which there are no drug or surgical answers."

Many holistic veterinary practitioners see themselves as educators who show their clients how to be more active partners in the health of their animals and how to nourish the natural healing intelligence that exists in all creatures. Before he passed away in 1999, Norman Ralston, DVM, of Mesquite, Texas, devoted a career spanning more than half a century to educating pet owners. "Alternative medicine is not just going to the doctor or veterinarian, getting a pill, and then going home and doing the same thing as before that got you or your animal in trouble," he used to say. "People appreciate it when they can begin to see results and realize that there are things they can do to make a difference."

No one approach—neither conventional, with its powerful drugs and sophisticated surgery, nor alternative with its less invasive, more natural "whole" body solutions—has all the answers. Increasing numbers of doctors and veterinarians believe that the future of medical practice lies in integrating the best and most effective techniques of both worlds. In this style of practice, doctors will use what works the best and is the least invasive or toxic. The choices will be vast: herbs, homeopathic remedies, vitamins, drugs, surgery, acupuncture, chiropractic, and magnet therapy, to name just a few modalities. Indeed, many of the veterinarians whose comments you will read in this book have developed this integrative approach long before the term "integrative" or "complementary" medicine became popular.

Personal health improvement starts with a commitment to eat better, exercise more, and handle the stress in our lives. Improving the health of companion animals also involves similar commitments on the part of the caregiver and starts with knowing our animals better. As was emphasized in the foreword to this book, there is no substitute for knowing our animals and watching for signs that may indicate a subtle shift in behavior, energy, and health, signs that may not even register on standard tests. If you feel there is a negative or unusual change in your cat, bring it to your veterinarian's attention.

THE INDIVIDUALITY FACTOR

The alternative approach strongly emphasizes the individuality of patients. Holistic practitioners assess each Being for unique physical and emotional clues in an attempt to restore systemic energy and balance. Ancient healing systems, such as Chinese and Ayurvedic medicine, are based on individualized treatment.

"In medical schools the emphasis is basically on getting rid of symptoms," says Mark Haverkos, DVM, of Oldenburg, Indiana. "Most of the time you treat the same symptom or disease in a hundred patients with the same medication or operation."

Haverkos says he began to think differently after a conversation years ago with Frank Fool's Crow, a widely respected Sioux medicine man.

"I wanted to know how he treated urinary tract infections with herbs," Haverkos recalls. "So I asked this great healer through an interpreter. Fool's Crow spoke very little English. The translator didn't do a good job in explaining what the urinary tract was. In the back-and-forth between us, I referred to 'making water.' The meaning now became clearer to the medicine man, but he had been around for too long to make a generality.

"His answer was: 'Whose water? Yours? Mine? A cat's? Which cat?'

"With that one comment the significance of individual treatment dawned on me, and I think I became a much less arrogant medical student," says Haverkos. "You can get really wonderful results from natural approaches to treat symptoms, but you may be able to go only to a certain level, because at some point in the healing of a Being you have to recognize the individuality of that animal and seek a health professional who can treat it individually."

A journal is one good way to keep track of your cat's health. Note down dates of moves, dramatic events in the household, veterinarian visits and prescriptions, and diet changes, all of which have the potential to cause reactions or behavioral or health problems. Observe your animal closely after treatments or vaccinations, which can create adverse reactions.

Ask your veterinarian to show you how to routinely check your animal's teeth, ears, eyes, and other body parts. Even while petting your animal, you can run your hand easily over the body in a search for any bumps, lumps, or anything abnormal.

The bottom line is this: Your cat is an individual just as you are. It has its own genetic blueprint and set of weaknesses, strengths, nutritional requirements, and reactions to medication or natural remedies. The more you know about your animal, the better you can carry out your responsibility as caregiver.

2

The Ill-Health Epidemic

"Do you see more serious disease among cats now than when you started in practice?"

I asked this question of every veterinarian interviewed for this book. Some of them have been practicing for half a century, most of them for twenty or more years. The status of cats, from their collective clinical perspective, is this:

- There are more chronic diseases.
- There are more animals with weakened immune systems and, as a result, more infections. "I am constantly treating chronic ear, urinary tract, and skin infections, situations where every scratch turns into a sore," says Joseph Demers, DVM, of Melbourne, Florida.
- There is more cancer. Some veterinarians speak in terms of an epidemic. They say their practices are inundated with cancer cases.
- There are more allergies.
- There are more skin problems. There is more itchy skin and severe disorders, and not just related to fleas.
- There is more tooth decay and periodontal disease.
- There are more serious conditions among young animals that were previously seen mostly among older animals.
- There are more middle-aged animals with the appearance and organs of old animals.

"Why is this so?" I asked the veterinarians. They cited combinations of the following:

- **Improper breeding practices.** Animals are bred today for looks, beauty, salability, and physical criteria to win show ribbons. "Kitty mills" then mass-produce the same designer cats. Such practices include inbreeding, where brothers and sisters, fathers and daughters, are bred with each other, and line breeding between cousins, grandparents, and grandchildren. Cats are being created with an emphasis on good looks rather than good health. This activity, ongoing for years, is perpetuating widespread genetic weaknesses and ill health. Each generation of cats appears to be potentially more susceptible to illness.

  "A genetic time bomb is going off at an earlier age, in all breeds, among animals being programmed for death and not for life," says Alfred Plechner, DVM, of Los Angeles.

  Young Abyssinians and Persians are plagued with tooth decay and periodontal disease. Persians often develop chronic upper-respiratory problems from breeding for a pushed-in face, which causes persistent eye discharge and constant snuffles. The anatomical deformity has undermined a first line of defense in the immune system. Maine Coons are predisposed to heart disease, which can strike down a cat at an early age.

  The genetic fallout of poor health is seen not only with purebreds, but increasingly even with mixed breeds from the pound or shelter. They are carrying the purebred defects in their blood, and they are being affected also. Similar problems are occurring among feral cats, the street cats that have a high rate of inbreeding within their own families. This creates the same kind of narrowing gene pooling that you see with purebreds.

- **Poor-quality, high-processed, and chemically preserved diet.** Veterinarians say they repeatedly treat problems related to food, such as skin, urinary tract, and cardiac disorders. In the wild, cats are not falling over dead with heart problems and urinary blockages.

- **Overvaccination.** The proliferation of vaccinations is a major problem. Vaccines trigger skin problems and other disorders and have been definitely linked to fibrosarcomas, aggressive cancers of the connective tissue that are intractable and resistant to treatment.

- **Too much medication.**

- **Environmental pollution.** Cats are very sensitive to the environment, to urban pollution, to pollen, and to the gasses emitted by a new carpet in the house. They have a delicate system that is finely tuned and balanced.

- **Stress.** Cats by nature are predators. A confined apartment existence may contribute to a variety of health problems.

The health status of cats, as described by this cross-section of veterinary clinicians, is not a pretty picture. It is, as Karen Bentley, DVM, of Guelph, Ontario, puts it, "a massive health mess." The commentaries from the veterinarians add up to a loud and clear wake-up call to pet owners to become smarter and better-informed caregivers.

3

The Problem with Pet Food

IF YOU ASK a holistic veterinarian how to improve the health of your cat, the first question he or she will ask you is this:

"What are you feeding your cat?"

As a group, holistic veterinarians are keenly interested in nutrition and diet. To them, food is a primary healing tool, "the mother of all natural remedies." Without good nutrition a pet cannot thrive. It won't be able to resist infections, fleas, or parasites. Medications and natural remedies won't work well.

The veterinarians I have interviewed are consistently critical of the quality of most commercial pet food. They doubt whether the overcooked, chemicalized, refined, and "scientifically formulated" products you buy can ever create radiant health or maintain a state of harmony in a cat. They are concerned that long-term feeding of inferior ingredients that are typically used in pet foods render animals toxic and disease-prone. Bill Pollak, DVM, of Fairfield, Iowa, says flatly: "The diseases we are treating is the food we are feeding."

Critics like Pollak point out that food has to be more than just the quantity of proteins, fat, carbohydrates, and added vitamins. It's the freshness, wholesomeness, energy, and digestibility of food that counts also. In these categories the veterinarians give failing grades to most commercial foods.

If this assessment comes as a surprise, then you need to know a little about the nature of the ingredients contained in the bags and cans you buy for your animals. The industry behind these products is big, big business—topping sales of $10 billion a year in the United

States alone. Competition is fierce among the major manufacturers. They try to win your allegiance with hundreds of millions of dollars in advertising, meaningless and misleading nutrition claims, and cute names for products. In this competitive scramble, however, quality and good nutrition are often sacrificed to economics and profit. Unfortunately there are no government standards regulating quality, which changes even within single product lines of a company as cheaper ingredients are constantly sought to replace more expensive ones.

If you think you are feeding the equivalent of sirloin steak out of those bags and cans, think again. The ingredients generally used are from sources unfit for human consumption. They include the following:

- **Meat.** Condemned and contaminated protein from slaughterhouses. Road-kill. Four-D livestock, meaning dead, diseased, disabled, and dying. And even euthanized companion animals—dogs and cats! These sources are rendered—that is, mixed together and "sterilized"—for use in subsequent processing into pet food. Many of the meat sources contain levels of drugs, hormones, and pesticides considered too high for safe human consumption.

- **Grains (carbohydrates).** Two of the top three ingredients listed on the labels of dry pet food (kibble) are generally some form of grain. They tend to be the cheap dregs from the human food chain. Frequently the grain is corn, such as ground yellow corn or corn gluten meal. Cats are true carnivores. They need meat. A diet high in corn, or any grain, makes no sense for a cat. But from the manufacturing standpoint, corn and other cereals being used to replace meat provide much cheaper and inferior protein sources than meat.

According to a 1996 report by the Animal Protection Institute of America, what you purchase and what the manufacturers advertise are two entirely different products. "The difference is threatening your animal's health, cutting short any chance of him enjoying old age, and maybe even killing him now," the report said. "The ingredients they are using are not wholesome, and the harsh manufacturing practices that make those nifty little shapes, the ones our companion animals surely love to eat, destroy what little nutritional value the food ever had."

The institute report described pet food manufacturers as "masters" in the art of taste enhancement—that is, getting animals to eat something "they would normally turn up their noses at." One way they do this is to spray kibble with discarded restaurant grease that has been stabilized with powerful chemical antioxidants. "Pet food scientists have discovered that animals love the taste of these sprayed fats," the report said. They want a food that animals will eat eagerly, and hopefully become addicted to, so that you return again and again to buy their product. Taste appeal, not quality, is paramount.

Many other chemical additives are used that increase the palatability, extend the shelf life, and improve the appearance so the product will look good enough to eat (but more important, will look good enough for you to buy). The pet food manufacturing process enlists some of the biggest names in chemical coloring of our time. Some of these dyes can actually make susceptible animals hyperactive. Sodium nitrite may be present to prevent fading of colors. Or Red Dye #40 may be used to create the appearance of a fresh, meaty look. Both these agents have long been linked to cancer or birth defects in laboratory animals and are even banned in some countries. Is color important to animals? Not as much as to you. The cosmetic effect is all for you—the buyer. Other chemical additives used to create an appealing finished product include anticaking, antimicrobial, coloring, firming, flavoring, drying, pH control, and surface finishing agents, and emulsifiers, sequestrants, synergists, texturizers, lubricants, and sweeteners.

PETS AS PET FOOD

You are probably not aware of the questionable nature of pet food. Why would you be? You are obviously interested in the well-being of your pet, but you also want to feed conveniently and inexpensively. So you purchase the commercial pet food that is readily available, assuming that it is good for your pet.

That is just what Ann Martin thought. Like most pet owners, she fed her household of animals—two dogs and four cats—with pet food she bought at the store. When the dogs became ill in 1990 after eating a popular commercial pet food, the Canadian woman had the food analyzed. The results disturbed her, and she started asking questions of people in the pet food industry and the government. The answers didn't satisfy her. So Martin set out on a personal fact-finding investigation of pet food that lasted seven years. Eventually, she put her experience and findings into a book that every pet owner should read: *Food Pets Die For—Shocking Facts About Pet Food* (New Sage Press, Troutdale, Oregon).

Martin says her investigation revealed that "just about anything and everything is fair game for use in pet food. Labels do not indicate the hidden hazards that lurk in most cans and bags." One of the most shocking practices she learned about was the use of euthanized pets as part of the rendered mix that goes into pet foods. Despite the denial by the industry that this is happening, says Martin, "dogs and cats from shelters, pounds, and even veterinary clinics are ending up in pet food. Some people seem to feel that this is not a problem; after all, dogs and cats are a source of protein. What they neglect to consider is that 90 percent of these animals have been treated with high levels of drugs prior to their demise. These drugs, antibiotics, hormones, and so on all withstand the rendering process and in fact can become more toxic. The companies selling the dyes and flavor enhancers are doing a landslide business, and as long as consumers are not offended by the smell and look of pet food, they assume it is a good quality."

In 1990 *San Francisco Chronicle* investigative reporter John Eckhouse brought this practice to public attention. He found that each year millions of dead American dogs and cats are processed along with billions of pounds of other animal materials into tallow and meat meal used for thousands of items, including cosmetics and pet food. The practice is not illegal and probably accounts for only a very small percentage of the protein content of pet food, Eckhouse reported. One veterinary official who confirmed the practice said that "when you read pet food labels and it says meat or bone meal, that's what it is—cooked and converted animals, including some dogs and cats."

Ann Martin once believed that she was buying quality. Now, her opinion is that "most pet food is garbage—unregulated garbage." Her animals now are fed only home-prepared food.

THE MOST HIGHLY PROCESSED FOOD ON THE PLANET?

The Animal Protection Institute report concluded that more than 95 percent of pets receive their nutritional needs from a single source—commercial pet food. This, then, is what most of our pets are eating—probably the most highly processed food on earth, where the magic of food technology sanitizes and camouflages the impurity of the product. Is there any wonder, holistic veterinarians ask, that chronic disease is so rampant?

Many animals are intolerant to the ingredients. This rejection is often expressed as violent illness or chronic health problems and often triggers a hypersensitivity and overreaction to flea and insect bites, pollens, soaps, sprays, and environmental contaminants. Dry food is a major offender because it is a concentrated collection of many of the foods that are the most allergenic for animals. Moreover, and particularly for cats, a constant ration of dry food is a sure invitation to health problems.

Holistic veterinarians say that commercial food just doesn't support organ function well. They frequently see cats that are middle-aged yet have the decrepit liver, kidneys, and other vital organs of very old animals, along with dry, lusterless skin.

If the pet food picture seems bleak, don't be discouraged. Read on. Increasingly, health-conscious consumers are demanding more quality. They are realizing that the food is causing many problems. Fortunately there is an industry response to this growing demand and awareness in the form of higher-quality products and more natural pet foods on the market. These, and other simple dietary options covered in the following chapters, will show you how to improve your cat's nutrition and prospects for better health.

4

Shifting to a Better Diet

FOR YEARS ALL of us have been hearing from experts about the importance of eating a better, more natural diet. We've been told that our hearts, arteries, bones, brains, and every moving part of the body benefits from healthy, wholesome food. The message of food's healing power is nothing new. More than 2,500 years ago, Hippocrates, regarded as the father of Western medicine, badgered his countrymen to "let thy food be thy medicine and thy medicine be thy food." This is timeless wisdom, totally relevant in today's age of fast food and rampant chronic disease.

The energy we call life animates the cells that make up our body and direct its countless biochemical functions. Foods are the fuel of life. Poor fuel makes for little momentum in life. Our bodies do not function well on poor-quality food, any more than a finely tuned automobile functions well on poor-quality gasoline. Many of the illnesses of people can be prevented or minimized through better nutrition. It's the same for our pets. Holistic veterinarians regard diet as the basis for health and treating any condition. It's the foundation. Everything else they do for an animal builds on this foundation. Get kittens started on the right fuel or deal with the fallout of feeding the wrong fuel in older cats, veterinarians repeatedly say.

What is good fuel? It's different for different species. Bees need pollen. Koala bears need eucalyptus leaves. Cats need meat. They are pure carnivores, with nutritional requirements and a specialized digestive system designed for consuming meat. The veterinarians I spoke to were adamant on this point—meat is king for cats, and the closer you come to a diet of raw, whole prey for cats, the less likely that poor nutrition becomes a cause of illness and a potential obstacle to cure.

VEGETARIAN CATS?

Meat is real cat food. It is unnatural for cats not to eat meat. Nature has created a unique digestive tract and specific physiological requirements for these animals. Even if you follow a healthy vegetarian lifestyle, please don't try to impose your dietary preference on a cat. You will only be causing harm. Veterinarians tell me that trying to make a cat a vegetarian is a bad decision. Something is missing from the diet. Animals don't grow right. Their fur doesn't look right. They constantly come down with respiratory illnesses. They will become anemic.

As Carvel Tiekert, DVM, says, "Cats were not designed as vegetarians. They are obligate carnivores. Who are people doing this for? The animals or themselves?"

Sharing living space intimately with indoor cats has perhaps caused many of us to lose track of what cats are really about— descendants of wild predators. Cats subsisted on unprocessed and uncooked prey such as rodents, birds, lizards, and even insects. They hunted for their food, devouring their prey completely, including all the organs and plant matter contained in the gut.

Today, most house cats aren't hunting and bringing down prey. So they have to count on us to provide their needs. Store-bought food, particularly dry food, may accommodate your convenience and your busy schedule, but for the cat it is a flagrant violation of nature. Even though domesticated cats have now been eating commercially prepared, highly processed foods for generations, veterinarians do not believe that the need for natural food has been lost. They believe instead that cats miss their natural diet and the proper balance of vital nutrients, fluids, and ingredients present in raw tissue. Much of the commercially prepared pet foods, even those made from the best ingredients, are heavily cooked, overprocessed, and missing many living, natural substances.

Any time the laws of nature are violated, suffering, stress, and disease result. You don't have to look much further than the unnatural quality of commercial pet food to understand why so many cats are getting sick and decrepit before their time. Holistic veterinarians generally don't believe cats can be truly healthy eating only commercial foods on a long-term basis.

You may be thinking that your cat seems to be fine and all you're doing is feeding it every day from the bag of food you buy at the supermarket. You may be right, because just as there are people who smoke, drink, and eat poorly and yet do not suffer from debilitating problems and die at one hundred, there are many resilient, long-lived animals who exist solely on commercial foods. Most animals, however, are hugely benefited by notching up the quality of their diet. The benefits show up as healthier cats with better appearance, more vitality, and fewer veterinary bills.

In this and the following two chapters you will learn how to notch up the quality of your cat's diet. The options are simple and practical and don't require a big effort. Choose an approach, recipe, or combination of ideas that fits into your schedule. You will be pleasantly surprised at how big a difference you can make with a minimum effort. Let's consider your options from the angle of what type of food you can and should feed your cat. Michele Yasson, DVM, of Rosendale, New York, has provided a compact overview of options for optimum feeding in the following perspective.

DR. YASSON'S CAT FOOD GUIDELINES

1. **Semimoist foods.** Don't even think about them. This is the equivalent of junk food.

2. **Dry foods (kibble).** Better, but still detrimental. All mammals are meant to eat fresh, whole natural foods, not dehydrated foods. Within this category, however, certainly the higher-quality natural brands are preferred (see chapter 5). Fortunately these are becoming more available, not only at health food stores, but also at general pet and feed supply outlets.

3. **Canned foods.** This is the minimal level of quality for healthy maintenance and for animals that need to do some healing.

4. **Fresh prepared foods.** The best choice, for them—and for us. The best rule of thumb that I know is as follows: Give half and even more as meat, preferably raw, the rest as vegetables and grain. Keep in mind that carnivores most often choose herbi-

vores (plant eaters) as their prey and eat their intestinal contents, which are predigested, or "cooked" vegetables. Many of my clients don't have the time to prepare meals for their pets. If an animal is seriously sick, there is no choice. If not, my recommendation is simple: Virtually anything you are eating that is healthy for you is healthy for your pets, so share liberally, up to 50 percent of the total volume of the diet. Make sure the added foods are provided in variety to avoid creating imbalances.

SIX STRATEGIES FOR IMPROVING THE DIET

Before introducing your options for improved feeding in the next chapter, let's now consider six important points:

1. How to switch the diet.

2. Adding meat—preferably raw.

3. Should you feed your cat grains?

4. Honor the individuality of your cat.

5. Feed the best you can without straining.

6. Preventive shopping—foods to avoid.

How to Switch the Diet

Cats, by nature, are suspicious about changes in their routine, and especially to changes in their diet. Introducing them to a new food, even if it is healthier, can be a major challenge once they have become habituated. Many animals become virtually "addicted" to a set diet. If you have a very persnickety cat, you are going to have to outfox it. The operative tactic any time you want to add anything to a cat's diet is stealth. Use the sneak attack. Start with a tiny amount of the food-to-be. Start low. Go slow. That's the only way to pull it off with a cat. If you put out a new food from one day to the next, most cats won't eat it. Or if they like it and eat it, they may develop diarrhea. Sudden changes may cause digestive upset, especially with the young and the old and also in cats with a tendency to gastrointestinal problems. Cats are very sensitive. Take your time.

The following ten-day plan suggested by Nancy Scanlan, DVM, works in many cases.

First four days	1/4 new food	3/4 old food
Next three days	1/2 new food	1/2 old food
Final three days	3/4 new food	1/4 old food

But you may want to go even slower for superfussy cats. If it takes two, three weeks or even more, it's worth the additional time to entice your cat to eat more wholesome food. Veterinarians say that even if they know an animal is eating a poor diet, they still go slow and don't make drastic changes.

Try to introduce variety when animals are young, before they are set in their eating ways. It's easier earlier in life than later. In many cases older cats won't accept changes.

Many people feed more than twice a day, which tends to make animals very picky. If fed twice, or better yet once a day, cats start to eat all sorts of foods. Skip a meal or two if your cat is basically healthy. A hungrier cat will be more receptive. Don't withhold food any longer than a couple of meals, however.

If your cat boycotts the change, as some may do, don't issue an ultimatum: "If you don't eat this, you starve!" Surrender. Go around it. You can find something tasty and nutritious. If their taste buds are set for one thing and you attempt to overpower them, you are wasting good time. Be flexible and creative. That's the key to success.

ADDING MEAT—PREFERABLY RAW

Many holistic veterinarians recommend raw food, and particularly raw meat, as a large part of a cat's regular diet. They say that feeding raw creates and sustains good health and also has the power to clear up many health problems for the large majority of animals. Digestive and skin problems improve rapidly, as do other deep-seated conditions. Very sick animals feel better and show renewed signs of vitality and energy.

Cats, of course, evolved on raw food, primarily raw meat. Raw foods contain their own built-in supply of enzymes, which facilitates the process of digestion. When food is cooked, the naturally occurring enzymes are destroyed, causing the body to activate its own enzymes to break down the food.

Advocates of raw meat frequently refer to the landmark research half a century ago of Francis M. Pottenger Jr., M.D., a California physician who raised cats for the purpose of studying allergic states and adrenal exhaustion. In his research he observed that cats eating cooked meat and heat-processed (pasteurized) milk experienced reproduction problems, deformed offspring, physical degeneration, and allergies that became progressively worse from one generation to the next. Pottenger then switched to raw meat and milk and witnessed a dramatic reversal in the health status of his cats. They reproduced with ease, were easier to handle, and had superior bone structure, shiny fur, and a general freedom from parasites and disease. Pottenger's research, from 1932 to 1942, involved more than nine hundred cats.

Veterinarians say you can give your cat anywhere from 50 to 90 percent of its food as raw meat. The recommended sources are turkey, rabbit, lamb, chicken, beef, venison, and fish. Don't use pork because of the risk of parasites.

What about the risk of bacterial contamination from raw meat? you may be thinking. We have all heard reports about humans becoming ill from eating tainted meat. Chicken, in particular, has been associated with pathogens such as E. coli and salmonella, and some animals have been known to develop mild diarrhea. The large majority of veterinarians I spoke to have been recommending raw meat for years without any problems. They say the benefits far outweigh the risks and that fears of feeding raw food usually disappear as the increased health of an animal becomes more evident. Cats, moreover, have strong stomach acids to counteract pathogens.

A number of veterinarians, however, did express reservations and suggest that people uncomfortable with the raw food concept should cook the meat slightly to minimize any potential danger. Steam or sauté the meat until the redness is gone. This practice may also be necessary for those animals who have lost the ability to digest raw meat after generations on cooked or commercial food and who may throw up or poorly absorb the nutrients.

Another option, if you have concerns over feeding raw meat, is to soak the meat in food-grade 3 percent hydrogen peroxide for 20 minutes. Use 1 tablespoon of peroxide in 1 pint of water. After soaking, rinse off with water and feed. Don't worry about any residual hydrogen peroxide, says Roger DeHaan, DVM, of Frazee, Minnesota. "A little bit can't hurt. In fact, it is helpful against yeast and any other parasites your animal may have."

If you choose to feed raw meat, the following guidelines from knowledgeable veterinarians will help you do it safely:

- As already mentioned, start low and go slow, particularly with older cats. You may, in fact, want to start with cooked meat and then transition slowly into raw meat. Or you may want to chop up the meat in the beginning and with time move to small chunks of raw meat. Some cats may regard raw meat, their natural food, as nonfood and reject it, or may eat only a small portion of it, while remaining ever addicted to their accustomed processed diet. To know your individual cat's level of acceptance, you'll simply have to test it. Many cats go immediately for the gusto of raw meat.

- Make sure the meat you serve is fresh.

- Don't use raw hamburger, which has more potential to collect bacteria.

- If you make a large batch of meals at one time, you may want to cut up the meat into daily portions and store them in plastic sandwich bags in the freezer. Take the next day's portion out of the freezer and place it in the refrigerator section for overnight thawing. When it is time to feed, put the bags with the meat in a glass or pot of warm water for a few minutes to warm the temperature of the meat. Keep the bags sealed so water doesn't seep into the meat.

- Use a clean fork or spoon to handle the meat. Don't use your hands.

- If the meat has an "off" odor or a questionable color, don't feed it.

- If you can afford it, and it is not a strain, organic is the highest quality. Organic meats do not contain the antibiotics and hormone residues present in commercially grown meats.

- Don't regard raw meat as kibble, which has been treated with preservatives. You can't fill your animal's feeding bowl with raw meat and then leave for work. Pick up what hasn't been eaten in fifteen or twenty minutes and toss it out. Then clean the dish. Also wash the utensils and any surface that has been in contact with the meat.

RAW MEAT AND PEOPLE'S ALLERGY CONNECTION?— CHRISTINA CHAMBREAU, DVM

I have found that allergies to cats clear up when you start feeding animals raw food. This was dramatically demonstrated to me in the case of a female veterinary technician who volunteered her services for a woman who ran a rescue facility for dozens of older cats. Normally, because of allergies to animals, the technician could not work around the animals for more than an hour at a time. The woman operating the facility decided at one point to switch the diet of her cats to primarily raw food. Within a period of two weeks the technician was able to stay for an entire day.

SHOULD YOU FEED YOUR CAT GRAINS?

Commercial dry foods for cats, and even many popular home-meal recipes, contain a sizable amount of grains as the source of carbohydrate. Currently, increasing numbers of holistic veterinarians are questioning whether animals should be eating so much grain. Many have found that some animals, no matter what their chronic problem is, seem to improve when grains are reduced or eliminated from the diet.

Let's say your cat is eating a diet based on 60 percent meat and 20 percent each of grains and vegetables, yet there is a persistent skin condition or some sign of less than optimum health. You may want to experiment by cutting out the grain and feeding just meat and some vegetables. If you see improvement, that indicates that your particular cat should be getting fewer grains or perhaps no grains at all.

Dr. Chambreau recalls the case of a cat who belonged to a veterinarian friend of hers. The cat, whose diet was 60 percent raw meat, had kidney problems. "My friend decided to try a 90 percent meat diet," she says. "On the new diet, the cat's kidney values all improved and its symptoms disappeared. There are many cats, and dogs as well, doing great eating no grains, just meat and vegetables."

Honor the Individuality of Your Cat

Don't lump all animals together. Each pet, like each of us, is an individual with individual tastes and reactions. One cat may prefer turkey over chicken. One may like steamed vegetables. Another may prefer them raw. Another may walk away from any vegetable. Try to determine your animal's individual needs and preferences. Always keep individuality and variety in mind as long as you don't forget quality.

Feed the Best You Can Without Straining

If your budget will allow it, feed organic food. This is the highest quality you can buy, for your health and your pet's. Cats are small, sensitive critters, at risk for accumulating the chemicals, hormones, and antibiotics present in commercial meat. Moreover, you may not want to support with your purchases the cruel, intensive-confinement practices used in modern meat-raising operations. While organic is the best from many angles, it is important to do what is affordable. Don't think that the only way to do it "right" is to feed organic, range-fed meat and organic vegetables. Straining for what is not easily obtained may cause stress and justification for stopping a more natural diet. Start from where you are and improve the level of nutrition for your pet comfortably. Don't forget the other vital things necessary for the health of your animals—the companionship, the exercise, and a nurturing environment. They all factor into the equation of health.

Preventive Shopping—Foods to Avoid

When buying any commercial food for your cat, read the label and avoid products with chemical preservatives, dyes, and additives. In particular, avoid the following:

- **Cheap, plain-wrapped "generic" pet food products.** It is probable they contain highly questionable ingredients and are often reject or substandard chows sold "out the back door" by major manufacturers. You get what you pay for. Poor-quality foods, fed over any length of time, are harmful for the health of your animal.

- **Semimoist foods.** These products appear red, moist, and pliable like real hamburger meat. They contain a full complement of sugar and chemical additives that you and I would avoid if we are truly interested in our health. They frequently cause allergic or allergiclike reactions and may contribute to pancreas or blood sugar problems.

- **"Lite" food.** It's a joke, full of empty calories and junk. Veterinarians say a cat will eat more of it than regular food and maintain the same weight or even put on weight.

HOW TO TELL IF YOUR CAT IS EATING A HEALTHY DIET

After you make changes to your cat's diet, you will want to monitor the results of your efforts. Canadian expert Edmund R. Dorosz, DVM, of Fort MacLeod, Alberta, author of *Let's Cook for Our Cat*, has compiled a simple method. It is based on evaluating three things: 1) your animal's appearance and condition; 2) behavior; and 3) stools.

SKIN — THE MOST IMMEDIATE SIGN

Skin is the largest organ in the body and offers a "quick read" of your pet's nutritional status. A dull hair coat and shedding are telltale signs of unhealthy skin below. If you part the hair, you will often find dry, flaky, and inflamed skin. This kind of a condition is associated with problems such as fleas, mites, ringworm, and inflammatory allergies. Max and Indy, my two cats, have lustrous hair coats because I feed them well, but if I have to leave town for a week or two, the cats receive commercial pet food. I feed them the best commercial food I can find; nevertheless I can tell the difference immediately. When I come back, the hair coat is dull and there is shedding all over the carpet.

BEHAVIOR

A cat receiving good nutrition is a happy, active, and responsive cat. Dullness, irritability, hyperactivity, nervousness, or restlessness can be caused by diet. Behavioral changes usually take several weeks to appear after the start of a new diet.

STOOLS

Most cats have one or two bowel movements daily. More may indicate a poor-quality diet. A proper diet and smooth-running digestive system produce a small amount of formed, brown firm stools. Liver or pancreas problems affect digestion and result in abnormal stools. Signs of a problem in the digestive tract include soft, loose, watery, light-colored or black, and smelly stools. If a cat doesn't have enough moisture, its stools will be dry and hard and may be difficult to pass. Medical attention should be sought if you see any of these signs.

DR. DOROSZ'S GOOD FOOD–BAD FOOD CHECKLIST

SIGNS	GOOD	BAD
Eyes	Bright, alert, clear	Dull, cloudy, tearing, red
Nose	Cool, moist, clean, soft	Hot, dry, hard
Teeth	Clean, white, shiny	Dirty, yellow, foul-smelling
Ears	Clean, dry	Inflamed, waxy, foul-smelling
Hair	Shiny, soft, clean	Dull, dry, dandruff, hair loss
Skin	Soft, pliable	Dry, greasy, inflamed, itchy
Muscles	Firm, developed, defined	Soft, lacking
Condition	Ribby (feel ribs)	Obese, potbelly, waddling walk
Paws	Smooth, resilient	Cracked, sore, nails brittle
Anus	Clean, dry	Inflamed, itchy anal glands
Urine	Light yellow, average volume	Dark or clear, large amounts

✵ 5 ✵

Feeding Option #1

ADDING MEAT AND TABLE SCRAPS TO A
QUALITY COMMERCIAL FOOD

WITH ONLY A minor effort and hardly a bite out of your time, this simple option gives you a powerful upgrade in the quality of the diet you feed your cat. The veterinarians I interviewed say that you really need to do at least this much and not rely solely on commercial pet food.

Here's what's involved:

- Feed the highest-quality pet food you can find and use that as the springboard, the base, for a better diet.
- To this base add a mix of fresh meat and vegetables. Add what you eat—if you yourself eat well. "Animals will be a whole lot healthier if a portion of their diet contains fresh and raw food," says Pamela Wood-Krzeminski, DVM, of Boca Raton, Florida.
- A pet multi-vitamin/mineral supplement, along with extra vitamin C.

THE RECOMMENDED BRANDS

To put this option into gear, purchase the best-quality commercial product you can find. What is the best on the market? Obviously you'll never know from the advertising claims. However, there are many premium brands and a number of so-called natural diets made by health-conscious manufacturers with higher-quality ingredients and few or no chemical additives. Your choices should be among these products.

Holistic veterinarians place a priority on nutrition. For that reason I asked each one I interviewed to name the pet food brands he or she recommends to clients. You will find the results of this informal survey below, with the brands most often mentioned listed first. The survey is hardly a scientific study of quality, but at least it gives you the preferences of nutritionally oriented veterinarians. The list includes telephone numbers of companies should you want information on products and where to purchase them.

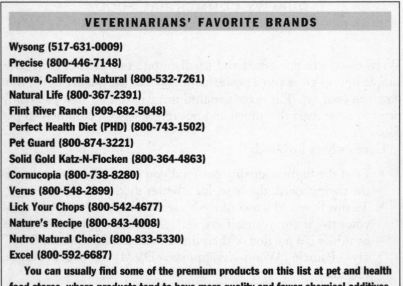

VETERINARIANS' FAVORITE BRANDS

Wysong (517-631-0009)
Precise (800-446-7148)
Innova, California Natural (800-532-7261)
Natural Life (800-367-2391)
Flint River Ranch (909-682-5048)
Perfect Health Diet (PHD) (800-743-1502)
Pet Guard (800-874-3221)
Solid Gold Katz-N-Flocken (800-364-4863)
Cornucopia (800-738-8280)
Verus (800-548-2899)
Lick Your Chops (800-542-4677)
Nature's Recipe (800-843-4008)
Nutro Natural Choice (800-833-5330)
Excel (800-592-6687)

You can usually find some of the premium products on this list at pet and health food stores, where products tend to have more quality and fewer chemical additives. Be sure to buy a product that turns over quickly and doesn't sit on the shelf for months. Some of the brands are not widely distributed to stores but can be sent to you via UPS or other commercial carriers.

Some of the veterinarians I spoke to were familiar with the owners, operations, and standards of some of these companies. But even if they knew a particular manufacturer and respected the company's efforts to ensure quality, they still recommended add-ons and rotating brands periodically.

They made the following points:

- The pet food industry is constantly changing. One company with a high-quality product now may start cheapening its food to save on cost, and soon it is not the same quality as before.
- Pet food manufacturers are not all-knowing, and something will probably be lacking in any commercial diet you give your pet.
- Many studies have cited health problems resulting from animals being fed a single product over a long period of time. To avoid the danger, select several brands and flavors that your animal likes, and rotate the foods. This provides pets with a variety of nutrient sources. You also reduce the chances of food intolerances and other disorders.

KIBBLE ALONE?—NOT A GOOD IDEA

Kibble is the ultimate convenience food. You open the bag and pour out a serving into the feeding bowl. But is your cat paying the price for your convenience? You bet, and a big price at that, if you are feeding it alone. Even if you feed good-quality, "natural" kibble, that by itself can be potentially harmful over time. I have been told repeatedly by veterinarians that many problems are eliminated by taking cats off dry food and feeding canned or, preferably, fresh meat instead. Such problems include feline urologic syndrome, skin disorders, arthritis, kidney failure, and constipation.

"If you go away for the weekend and you put out a bowl of kibble, you know your animal won't starve," says Jean Hofve, DVM. "Kibble is fine for that. But cats absolutely need wet food—and lots of it."

Cats originally were desert animals. Their kidneys were designed to be extremely efficient in order to conserve water. Historically they ate a fresh food diet of prey containing 70 percent body fluids. Kibble is a mere 5 to 10 percent moisture. Thus, a cat's kidneys are going to be overworked for an entire lifetime if you feed just kibble.

"I have seen kidney failure in cats four or five years old, and that is really upsetting," says Hofve. "It's different if the cat is seventeen or eighteen years old. But there is no excuse for this in young cats. These animals must have a wet diet. It protects their kidneys."

Another way to look at the pitfalls of kibble is through the perspective of Chinese medicine, where the continual consumption of "dry foods" is seen leading to "internal heat." The effect of this heating-up process on the organs is explained by Joseph Demers, DVM, who uses acupuncture and Chinese medicine in his Florida practice: "The animal on a diet of dehydrated food becomes dehydrated. The body builds up a lot of heat, which needs to be eliminated. Eventually you see burping, throwing up of bile in the morning, and upset stomachs. You see thick saliva, dry stools, and an animal panting after its evening meal even though the surroundings are cool."

Demers treats many animals suffering with the side effects of kibble. "I relate kibble to macaroni or rice you would take from the box and eat without cooking it," he says. "It is too dry, too processed, with too many chemicals. It contributes to chronic disease."

If circumstances necessitate that you feed kibble, you *must* add meat for the sake of your cat.

EASY UPGRADES

The following practical suggestions provide easy-to-do ideas for diet upgrades and variety using a higher-quality commercial food as a base. This option introduces "live food" into the diet with less reliance on overcooked, processed products.

The Three-Minute Plan—Robert Goldstein, VMD

I have many clients who spend hours preparing recipes for their animals. But they aren't the majority, so I try to focus on people who don't have much time, who tell me basically this: "I have three minutes and then I have to go to work. What can I do? I want the maximum protection for my cat in that period."

Here's what you can do in three minutes:

• Use any of the following of my favorite dry cat foods as a base:

Cornucopia, Lick Your Chops, Natural Life Cat, Sold Gold Katz-N-Flocken, or Wysong Cat.

- For added protein, use an already cooked, broiled rotisserie chicken (remove the skin and bones before feeding), cooked turkey breast, low-fat plain yogurt, low-fat cottage cheese, or a fertile egg yolk. Use organic if possible. The largest quantitative replacement of your base food for cats should be protein. Meat items can take the place of about one-quarter of your dry food; yogurt or cottage cheese, 15 percent. You can also use high-quality canned pet foods as a source for added protein. The brands I rate highest are Wysong, Lick Your Chops, Cornucopia, Natural Life, PetGuard, Precise, and Innova.

- For carbohydrates, add a palatable portion of whole grains such as brown rice, oatmeal, or millet. They are rich in B vitamins and fiber to help keep the intestinal tract clean. If you don't have time to prepare or cook a meal, reach for a packet of "quick cook" oatmeal, which retains much of its nutrients and fiber sources even in instant form. For speed you can use a parboiled brown rice, available in health food stores. Many animals are allergic to gluten, the concentrated protein fraction found in wheat. Millet is gluten-free, making it a good choice for hypoallergenic diets. Cats enjoy the taste of millet.

- Grated organic carrots and finely chopped broccoli are healthy additions. Cats also love zucchini, cooked or raw. Sprouts are a good source of "green," living foods, rich in chlorophyll, nature's elixir, which helps cleanse the blood. Sprinkle 1 teaspoon onto the food. Wheatgrass also provides healthy, concentrated nutrients. Start with 1 teaspoon of chopped wheatgrass and work up slowly to 1 tablespoon per meal. Avoid tomatoes; they are too acidic.

- Add a good cold-pressed oil such as olive or flaxseed. Use a virgin olive oil for the oleic fatty acid that will promote energy and skin conditioning. If your cat is prone to inflammatory conditions such as chronic skin problems, use flaxseed oil, which is high in the essential fatty acids linolenic and alpha-linoleic acids. Look for organic flaxseed products in dark containers, as this oil is quite fragile and will break down when exposed to light and heat. Store in the refrigerator. Add 1 teaspoon of oil and mix into the food.

• Add a vitamin and mineral supplement. I suggest Daily Health Nuggets, available through Earth Animal (800-711-2292), or Dr. Goodpet's Maximum Protection Formula (800-222-9932).

• Start slowly with this or any new diet program. Begin with small amounts and work your way up. If your cat consumes a large amount of vegetables that the digestive tract isn't accustomed to, loose stools or gas may develop. If this happens, just slow down. Feed less and increase more slowly. And don't forget fruit. Many cats like them, particularly melon. But no citrus; it's too acidic.

Organ Meat, Veggies, Yogurt, Add-Ons—Roger DeHaan, DVM

Wild cats don't go first for the muscle meat—they prefer the organs and stomach contents. Fresh, raw organ meats—heart, liver, and kidney—are alive with enzymes, hormones, and other growth factors, vitality and nutrition that can't be duplicated in a can.

Add some vegetables daily. Stomach contents are basically steamed, predigested, enzymatically processed herbs and vegetables. You don't need much: 1 tablespoon is enough. Start cats on the vegetable habit at a young age. You usually won't get fifteen-year-old cats to start eating vegetables. My preferences are carrots, broccoli, beets, green beans, alfalfa sprouts, and dark green leafy vegetables.

Yogurt is an excellent add-on. Give 1 tablespoon twice to five times a week.

Feed 1 egg or egg yolk twice a week.

The Liver "Remedy"—Edmund Dorosz, DVM

I regard liver as "nature's miracle food," rich in vitamins, minerals, fatty acids, and protein. Adding raw liver to your animal's regular diet is a simple step that yields major head-to-tail health benefits. You frequently see skin conditions improve just by supplementing the diet with liver. Feed 1 tablespoon a day or 2 to 3 ounces a week.

Some people refrain from eating or feeding liver because they believe that this organ is filled with toxins and other undesirable substances. Yes, it is the organ that filters out undesirables, but unlike the oil filter in our cars, the liver is a dynamic organ. The car filter retains the impurities. The dynamic liver filters them out and expels them.

Liver is a very nutritious food for us to eat and give to our animals.

Partially Raw Diet—Thomas Van Cise, DVM

I consistently see good responses to a simple, partially raw diet. Try to use organic products, if possible, as they have the highest quality.

Ingredients:

One-third as raw meat, such as beef, chicken, or turkey. The meat you choose depends on your pet's tolerance and preference for a particular food.

One-third as lightly steamed or blanched grated vegetables, such as carrots, squash, beans, and greens such as spinach and bok choy. This makes the vegetables more digestible without destroying nutrients and enzymes through cooking.

One-third as European-Style Cat Food Mix, made by Sojourner Farms (888-TO-SOJOS). This wholesome human-quality preparation contains nuts, grains, wheat germ, buttermilk powder, and dried kelp and is meant to be served with raw meat for a fully balanced diet. The food should be soaked for a few minutes before using to make it more digestible.

Partially Raw Diet #2—Carvel Tiekert, DVM

While I consider Precise, Natural Life, and Verus to be high-quality commercial foods, maybe as good as you can buy in processed foods, they are still processed. The enzymes and other natural factors that are alive in whole, raw foods have been killed in any commercially prepared food. For this reason I recommend supplementing the diet with raw meat.

I like fresh chunk beef, the cheapest stew meat you can find. Cut up the meat and freeze the pieces in plastic bags. I prefer that over hamburger, because when you grind up hamburger you take whatever bacteria there is on the outside and mix it into the inside. You damage the cells more. And if you let it sit in your refrigerator, you know what happens to it.

My real preference is for raw chicken necks or the raw tip section of chicken wings. This will provide raw meat and fat, a good source of calcium, and probably the next best thing to brushing for tooth and gum health. Chicken gizzards are also good. Cats require fats as an energy source, so don't skin the fat off the necks. Feed it skin and all. Give your animal about 1/2 to 1 ounce daily.

While I have not personally seen any health problems caused by supplementing the diet with raw chicken, there is nevertheless a risk of a bacterial contamination in poultry. I feel, however, that the risk-benefit ratio still favors the feeding of raw meat.

I also recommend vegetables, lightly steamed, and all the cat will eat. Older cats are difficult to get to eat vegetables, so try many different kinds. Try buttering the vegetables as an enticement. If younger cats are started on vegetables, they will often eat them.

A good general vitamin/mineral is always a good idea. My favorite product is NuCat (from Vetri-Science, 800-882-9993, available through veterinarians). I also recommend extra vitamin C in the amount of 250 milligrams a day. I prefer the sodium ascorbate powder form of vitamin C, which is easy to mix right into the food and is palatable for most cats.

TABLE SCRAPS: WHAT TO FEED, WHAT NOT TO FEED

Many veterinarians put down the idea of table scraps. But not the ones I talked to. Table scraps have gotten a bad rep because they supposedly upset the nutritional balance of "scientifically formulated" pet foods. If commercial diets are so scientific, why are so many pets sick and overweight? More likely the real reason for dissuading consumers to refrain from table scraps is that the pet food industry will sell less pet food.

Holistic veterinarians generally favor table scraps, as long as you keep them wholesome and simple. One commonsense guideline offered by Norman Ralston, DVM, is this: "If the food on your plate is harmful for your pet to eat, maybe you should not eat it yourself."

Here are the veterinarians' suggestions:

- Share a little of what you are eating every day with your pet. That provides taste and nutritional variety.
- Remember that all cats are individuals with individual tastes, sensitivities, and needs. Make sure what you're feeding is not causing allergic reactions.
- The volume of dry (commercial) food you normally feed should be lessened by the volume of table scraps you add.
- The digestive tract of the cat is geared for simpler food than we eat. Rich foods like ham, sauces, and cheese are invitations for trouble.
- Don't feed leftover fat and remnants that may not be healthy. No bacon or bacon grease. Besides the high levels of nitrites, the high heat used in cooking bacon creates many other unhealthful compounds. It is best not to use any fat drippings.
- Raw or steamed vegetables are excellent, particularly carrots, anything in the broccoli family, squash, and leafy greens. Many cats love the taste of cooked squash. Raw vegetables in general should be mashed, grated, or aged. Vegetables can be pureed in a blender, then left to sit in a container for a day or two before feeding.
- Try different fruit, particularly in hot summer months.
- Seaweed is a magnificent source of trace minerals. You will be surprised to know that many cats enjoy the taste. Just a tiny amount added to the regular diet can provide minerals that are missing from commercial diets. Nori, the black, thin seaweed used in sushi, has a fishy flavor that cats like.
- Stay away from spicy, salty, and fried foods. Unfortunately some animals can get addicted to such fare. No spicy chili, pepperoni, or luncheon meats.
- No sweets, cookies, or cakes.
- Store your leftovers in a plastic container with a tight cover and refrigerate. Use a bit at a time for flavor enhancing. Warm up the leftovers a bit after taking out a portion from the fridge.

✹ 6 ✹

Feeding Option #2

THE DELUXE TREATMENT: EASY-TO-MAKE
HOMEMADE MEALS

THERE'S NOTHING LIKE home cooking. For pets, too. Veterinarians have repeatedly told me that nothing works as well to create radiant and long-lasting health than fresh food prepared at home. People who eat this way themselves and who extend their efforts somewhat to include their animals have thriving pets who consistently look better than animals eating any store-bought food.

"The best and most inexpensive food you can feed your pet is food you prepare yourself," says Carolyn Blakey, DVM, of Richmond, Indiana, summing up a consensus opinion among holistic veterinarians.

So if you have the inclination, this chapter will show you how to go all out for your cat. You will be surprised how little time and effort it takes to prepare healthy meals. In fact, there isn't much cooking involved at all if you use raw meat.

Here are the basic guidelines:

1. Don't get fancy.

2. Keep the diet simple with fresh and varied foods. Rotate foods frequently.

3. Cats need meat and lots of it in their diet. Ideally the meat should be raw or lightly cooked. In the recipes below, the recommendations for the meat portion of the diet start at 50 percent and go as high as 90 percent.

4. Find a formula that works well for you and your animal.

5. Add a good pet multi-vitamin/mineral supplement to help achieve optimum nutritional intake, and consider extra vitamin C for keeping the immune system strong. Calcium and taurine should be added to homemade meals (see "Easy Cat" Recipe, following).

If you have any doubts about how your animal is doing on the diet, refer to the checklist of nutritional status signs at the end of chapter 4. To learn more about home-prepared meals, refer to the list of excellent books in appendix C. Better yet, consult with a nutritionally oriented holistic veterinarian who can individualize a program for your particular cat.

FEEDING WITH LOVE—NORMAN C. RALSTON, DVM

By putting your own love and energy into the food, you strengthen the relationship with your pet. This, of course, is the key to macrobiotic cooking. No amount of store-bought food, however natural, and of whatever quality, can give that kind of love. Food prepared fresh each day with love is special. It carries a special vibration, and the person or animal who eats it absorbs that energy. The effects on your pet's health will be impressive.

The "Easy Cat Diet"—Jean Hofve, DVM

Copy the natural diet as much as possible. A balanced diet including raw meat is thus the way to go for most cats. Proper hygiene and meat-handling procedures should always be observed (see discussion on raw meat in chapter 4). The exceptions to a diet with raw meat are immune-compromised animals, the very young, the very old, or any cat whose health status is uncertain. In addition, owners who are pregnant, undergoing chemotherapy treatment, or otherwise immune depressed should not handle raw meats at all. Cooked meats carry less risk of parasites and infectious organisms. Meat must be prefrozen to reduce the potential for some common infectious organisms.

Once a week you can include some kidney or liver. Organic only, however, especially the liver.

Cats eat whatever of a vegetable nature is present in the digestive tract of the prey they kill and eat. They will also eat a bit of grass. But that's about it for vegetables. Finely chop the vegetables, or use a blender or food processor to pulverize them. You can also lightly steam them. A tablespoon or two per pound of meat is adequate.

Grains are purely optional, and some experts suggest eliminating them from a cat's diet completely.

You must add calcium to a homemade meal. Figure about 500 milligrams per 100 grams (3 ounces) of meat, or about 1 to 2 tablespoons of human-grade bone meal per pound of meat. I recommend bone meal as a good source of calcium and use Bone All from Schiff, available in health food stores. Vitamins, minerals, and other micronutrients must be added to balance the diet. Celeste Yarnall, a breeder and cat nutritionist, has developed a number of good supplements intended to simplify and augment homemade diets. You provide the fresh ingredients—the meat, the veggies, and, if you choose to use them, grains—and then add the supplements fresh at feeding time. This is a good way to go if you're chronically short of time and energy, and who isn't? (For information on Yarnall's products, call 1-888-CEL PETS, or see her Web site at www.celestialpets.com.)

"Easy Cat" Recipe

Choose one of the following protein sources. Rotate proteins frequently, so the cat gets used to a variety of tastes.

    6 ounces ground turkey
    1/2 pound boneless chicken breast
    1/2 pound lean ground beef
    1/2 pound lean ground lamb
    1/2 pound beef, chicken, or turkey heart, ground
    Optional: once a week, substitute 4 ounces organic liver for
    one-half of any meat source

Mix your protein choice with the following:

1 to 2 tablespoons pureed vegetables or vegetable baby food (if you use baby food, be sure it has no onion powder, which is harmful to cats)

1 hard-boiled egg, chopped

2 teaspoons canola oil (or 1 teaspoon canola and 1 teaspoon flaxseed oil)

1/2 rounded tablespoon bone meal (Schiff's Bone All, available in health food stores) or 3 human-grade bone meal tablets, powdered

1/3 of a 250-milligram taurine tablet or capsule (about 80 milligrams), or 1/2 ounce chopped clams in juice (Taurine is an amino acid—a building block of protein—that cats need to obtain in their diet. It is contained in most meat and fish. In the past, many health problems have been attributed to taurine deficiency, particularly in commercial foods. As insurance, it is a good idea to supplement the diet with taurine.)

Directions: Make your meals in a batch—for instance, three pounds at a time. Combine the meat, oil, and bone meal, plus any veggies or grains, and freeze in meal-size portions. Thaw a daily ration the morning before. Mix in the other elements fresh at mealtime. Meat can be cut into chunks, but ground meat may be easier to handle. Grind vitamin, bone meal, and taurine tablets to a powder with mortar and pestle, blender, or coffee or nut grinder. Make sure any cooked items are cool before adding supplements. Feed an adult cat as much as it will eat in twenty minutes. Refrigerate leftovers promptly. Dump any raw meat left over. Feed adults twice a day. Kittens between two and four months old should be fed three to four times daily.

The Natural Raw Meat Diet—William Pollak, DVM

Start your pets on this type of diet slowly. An animal transitioning from a previous all-commercial food diet may have severely weak digestion. A water fast of one or two days can ease the transition. Follow the fast first with the meat portion of the diet for several days, then add the vegetables (for two more days), and then the grain portion, if you use grains. This will reduce the occasional side effects of diarrhea arising from too much internal purification occurring from the new diet (see Pollak's comments in box, "Be Alert for Healing Episodes").

Ingredients:

Protein: 75 to 90 percent raw meat. Use turkey, chicken, lamb, venison, beef, and fresh fish. Begin with chopped meat and fish. Larger pieces can be given after six to twelve weeks if desired. For convenience, it is okay to serve the same meat for three to four days. Then switch, if possible. Steady feeding of the same food can lead to sensitivities. If you have reservations about raw meat, know that you are cooking the meat to please yourself, not your cat. If that's the case, cook the meat as little as possible until you feel more comfortable. For people who have a block about feeding raw food, I recommend Perfect Health Diet (800-743-1502), an additive-free pet food that offers a high standard of quality and freshness. Eggs are an excellent source of protein. Feed one or two eggs twice weekly, depending on the size of the cat. Raw is fine with the shells broken into small pieces, or lightly scramble the eggs with butter. Pasteurized cow's milk can cause diarrhea, gas, and discomfort in less vital cats. Cottage cheese or cultured dairy products are usually okay. Raw milk (goat milk is best) can be well tolerated if introduced slowly into the diet once the cat has become accustomed to raw meat.

Vegetables: 10 to 25 percent raw, grated, or chopped. Use whatever is fresh at the grocery. Dark green leafy veggies, cauliflower, string beans, broccoli, zucchini, carrots, and turnips are good choices. I have found that cats will often sit and chew on carrots. Raw vegetables are the best. You may, however, have to lightly steam vegetables to get some cats to start eating them.

Grains: 0 to 5 percent. Cooked rye, millet, couscous, quinoa, buckwheat, and wheat are all fine. Cats have short, small digestive systems that can easily be overloaded. If your cat goes for it, share a small amount of cooked grain you yourself eat. You may want to add butter to help it go down.

Fats: Adding some cold-processed olive oil, sesame oil, butter, ghee (clarified butter), or canola is beneficial. These are sources of healthy fat. Give 1/8 to 1/4 teaspoon. Try varying the amounts to allow your cat to tell you what it desires.

Nutritional supplements: Use a multi-vitamin/mineral formula for cats, human-quality bone meal, colloidal minerals or kelp, and extra vitamins C and E. Start off in small amounts until the animal gets accustomed to the new tastes.

Directions: For convenience, mix up ingredients weekly. Freeze mixtures in containers or sandwich bags, and thaw portions in the refrigerator overnight that you will be using the next day. Add supplements at time of feeding.

How to Feed: Feed adult cats once a day. They will generally eat between 1/2 and 3/4 cup of food. In the beginning they may consume more food as their body attempts to compensate for nutritional deficiencies. Amounts will vary with activity, age, and digestive ability. Generally speaking, they will eat less than the normal amount of commercial food previously eaten. Don't be concerned. An animal doesn't need a lot of food if what it eats is quality. Today, animals on most commercial diets are simply being overloaded with excess amounts of low-quality food—with a disastrous impact on the organs. The best way to know whether you are feeding too much or not enough is to consider how your cat looks and acts. A "doughy" appearance is replaced by a more compact, solid conformation. There is less voracious feeding behavior. The eyes become bright and clear. There is overall greater energy and vibrancy, more calmness and responsiveness. There is almost always less drinking, with less urination and stool. This is natural. These characteristics become more prominent as higher-quality nutrition saturates the cells of the pet, a process that can take weeks to months. If more weight is needed, increase the food ration, adding both fat (or oil) or more meat.

Kittens and lactating and pregnant cats require more frequent feedings and slightly higher protein, fat, mineral, and dairy content in the diet. Dairy in the form of raw (unpasteurized) goat's milk is best, though not always necessary. Check to see that no diarrhea ensues.

BE ALERT FOR HEALING EPISODES— WILLIAM POLLAK, DVM

Some 15 to 20 percent of animals develop a "healing episode" as a result of purification of the system brought on by purer and more nutritious food. This may manifest in such transient symptoms as diarrhea or skin sores. The body is simply expelling accumulated impurities. This situation is, in a sense, a transition to a higher state of balanced health. The frequency, intensity, and duration of such episodes is totally dependent on an individual animal's health, nutritional state, age, and breed. As long as the animal is clear-eyed, bright, and full of the energy of life, these periods (should there be any) will quickly pass. The need for medical intervention is rare (for more details on feeding a raw diet, see Pollak's Web site at www.healthyvet.com).

V.J.'s Recipe—Mark Haverkos, DVM

The late V. J. Keating, DVM, a pioneer of holistic veterinary medicine who practiced in Oregon for many years, always recommended that you try to simulate what the animals naturally eat in the wilds. This, he felt, boosts the life force of pets and increases their level of health. I have applied this concept to my patients, and it has worked well. His basic formula was simple: up to one-half protein (meat) and one-quarter each of carbohydrates and vegetables.

The protein should be from the normal game range if possible: turkey, chicken, rabbit, and fish.

For the carbohydrates, brown rice.

For vegetables, any that the cat will eat.

The meat can be either raw or cooked. Mix with cooked vegetables and rice.

The "Time-Saver Recipe"—Karen Bentley, DVM

Time is the great dictator of how much effort you can put into a meal. I am often pressed for time, so years ago I developed a simple recipe that accommodates both time and nutrition. It is easy to put together and is nutritionally sound. It has served well for me and my busy clients for fifteen years and allowed us to conveniently provide quality nutrition to our animals.

Ingredients:
1 pound cooked chicken or raw beef
2 pounds frozen mixed vegetables
1 pound tofu
28 ounces pumpkin pie filling, a good source of fiber; cats like the taste!

Directions: Batch-mix and freeze into small containers. Feed 1 to 2 heaping tablespoons twice daily, depending on the size of the cat. At time of feeding, add the following supplements:

- Taurine, 250 milligrams daily. You can crunch tablets and mix into food.
- A multi-vitamin/mineral supplement such as Maximum Protection Formula, from Dr. Goodpet (800-222-9932), or Mega-C Plus, from Orthomolecular Specialties (408-227-9334). Follow label instructions.

The 1-2-3 Recipe—Carolyn Blakey, DVM

This recipe is as simple as 1-2-3. Just feed the following proportions of the three major food groups:

One-half or more of the mix as high-quality proteins—namely, real meat, and some of it raw if your animal will eat it.

Up to one-fourth as vegetables or fruits (lightly steam or grate the veggies).

Up to one-fourth as cooked whole grains (such as brown rice and oatmeal).

Be sure to add a good vitamin/mineral supplement and a digestive enzyme to the food before feeding to ensure that all the nutrients the animal needs are present and are well absorbed.

The only pet food I would add to this mixture this is European-Style Cat Food Mix, made by Sojourner Farms (888-TO-SOJOS). This blend of human-quality grains, herbs, dried sea vegetables, and ground nuts is very easy to prepare and adds solid nutrition.

Simple, Fresh, and Varied—Norman C. Ralston, DVM

The diet can be very simple. The important thing is to use fresh ingredients. Fresh doesn't mean expensive. Use a simple rule of thumb for proportions and vary ingredients according to your situation, availability, nutritional need, season, and weather. For animals, as well as for humans, variety is the key to staying on the diet.

Tailor the diet to your animal's particular needs. Some individual ingredients work better or are more palatable for one animal than another. That is something you can find out only by trial and error with your animals.

My cat Fulton, for instance, eats green beans, okra, and leafy green vegetables of different kinds. He loves cantaloupe. If I am eating melon, he has to have some also. He eats brown rice and squash. But that's my particular cat.

Here are general guidelines I have found particularly good for cats:

One-half of the diet is animal protein, just slightly cooked. Fish is my favorite recommendation. Cats love fish, then rabbit, followed by chicken and beef.

One-fourth as fresh vegetables, such as steamed squash, carrots, and broccoli. Blend or chop into small particles. I routinely recommend feeding squash, particularly yellow squash, to cats. Many cats love squash (of course, not all). I have one cat who won't eat squash if you starve him to death. If possible, choose vegetables in season and grown in the region where you live.

One-fourth as grain (brown rice, corn, barley, buckwheat, amaranth, millet, wheat). Be sure to cook the grains thoroughly and then blend them or run them through a food processor. That will enhance digestibility. Animals tend to gulp food down. Cats, by the way, seem to enjoy barley soup. Try it—add a little to their food for variety.

Seaweed, such as kelp or dulse, provides an excellent source of health-giving trace minerals. Add a pinch of powdered kelp. It contains six times as much calcium as cow's milk. Although it is expensive, cats seem to love nori, another seaweed; it smells like fish. Roast it a little, crumble it, and sprinkle it onto, or mix into, food.

WATER—CATS NEED IT, TOO

Cats are equipped to concentrate urine and conserve water, an inheritance from their desert ancestors. Their evolutionary beverage consisted primarily of the fluids in the natural prey they consumed. A domestic cat may not consume much water—perhaps a few sips a week—if it is on a diet emphasizing fresh, raw food, or canned commercial food with a high moisture content. Dry cat food, however, has only a slight amount of moisture. In any case, fresh water should always be available, no matter what kind of food the cat is eating. Preferably use filtered water. Tap water is full of chemicals and contaminants. Keep the drinking bowl clean and clear of any soap residue. Severe dehydration can occur in association with sickness such as fever and diarrhea. Young kittens are especially vulnerable, so be sure to monitor them closely if they become sick. One sign of a cat developing diabetes is an unquenchable thirst. Increased water consumption may also be a primary symptom of liver, kidney, and thyroid disease. Be alert to this telltale sign in any cat, but especially if you have an older cat.

THE BONE CONNECTION

Many people give their cats raw bones without any problem. Don't overdo it, however. If large quantities of bones are consumed, the pieces may compact into a mass and cause constipation. Particularly troublesome are pork bones, which are brittle and splinter easily. Stay away from pork altogether; it can make cats sick.

Cooked bones tend to splinter and might damage the gums. Some people recommend crunching cooked bones into crumbs and adding them to the food. The problem is that you might miss a piece, which can possibly cause some damage in the system.

7

Nutritional Supplements

FOR MORE THAN twenty-five years San Jose veterinarian Wendell Belfield, DVM, has routinely prescribed vitamins and minerals for his small animal patients. And for years many mainstream veterinarians and researchers dismissed the practice, particularly his aggressive use of vitamin C. Belfield has ignored his critics for the simple reason, as he says, "that the supplements work and make a big impact against disease."

Among dogs, for instance, he found that hip dysplasia, a crippling condition that leads to arthritis, could be prevented by a nutritional approach emphasizing sodium ascorbate, a nonacidic form of vitamin C. He has used a similar approach to turn negative hundreds of cats who previously tested positive for feline leukemia. Cats with signs of chronic illness improve. Queens with a history of infertility, abortions, or fetal resorption give birth to normal, healthy litters. Fading kitten syndrome is eliminated.

The reigning belief in veterinary thinking is that dogs and cats don't need extra vitamin C, because they produce the substance in the liver, unlike humans and guinea pigs, who do not, and who must obtain it in their diet or suffer a deadly condition called scurvy. Through his research and clinical investigations, Belfield found that dogs and cats were, in fact, poor producers of vitamin C compared with most other mammals and that they thrived when supplemented with the vitamin. His pioneering work has influenced a whole generation of nutritionally minded practitioners. They now routinely advocate vitamin C, and other supplements, in the treatment of disease and in general for optimizing the health of their animal patients.

Before 1990 vitamins and minerals were viewed narrowly by the medical establishment as vital elements in food that prevented certain nutritional deficiency diseases—such as scurvy. The mainstream attitude was that supplementation was unnecessary—and a waste of money—because a balanced diet provided you with all the good nutrition your body needed. For decades only a small minority of nutrition doctors vociferously contradicted this position and advocated supplements as a potent, safe, and inexpensive way to help treat illness and create optimum health.

Reality, along with a massive volume of research, has set the record straight. Surveys show that huge numbers of people fail to eat anything closely resembling a balanced diet. Moreover, much of the food that reaches our tables these days is grown on soil depleted by intense commercial farming and agrochemical practices. Many studies now show that individual nutrients at doses higher than those usually present in the diet can have a profound preventive and therapeutic impact on cancer, heart disease, and other serious illnesses.

Among our pets there is a crisis of health that parallels the human predicament. The mirage of the balanced diet is promoted by the pet food industry in the form of so-called complete and balanced diets. Ideally pets should get all the nutrients they need in food, but standard pet food sources are highly questionable, and the end products are usually low in freshness and high in additives.

The pet food industry generally serves up minimum amounts of nutrients designed to maintain adequate health. But today the contamination of the environment and the chemical additives in many commercial pet diets lessen the likelihood that minimum nutrition will maintain good health. Animals will survive on this food but never be really healthy, holistic veterinarians say.

"We need more nutrients provided by supplementation if we are to raise our animals to the level of optimum health and also sustain them through the stresses of pregnancy and disease," says Belfield.

Cats genuinely benefit from many of the same nutritional supplements that we humans take—vitamins, minerals, essential fatty acids (oils), digestive enzymes, and amino acids. The more removed animals are from natural diets, the more they need supplements. But even with solid homemade meals or a better commercial food, they tend to thrive that much more with supplements. Veterinarians report dramatic changes in cats after supplementation is started. Shaggy hair coats become lustrous. Health and vitality soar.

HOW TO CHOOSE THE RIGHT SUPPLEMENTS FOR YOUR CAT

What supplements should you use? The marketplace offers a dazzling multitude of products. Trying to find the right one for your pet can be confusing.

Your best bet is to find a nutritionally oriented practitioner to structure the most effective supplementation program for your cat based on its individual health status, age, diet, and stress level. Different conditions benefit from different supplements that require an expert's know-how.

There is another good reason to seek professional guidance: You don't want to overdo it. "I have had clients come in with shopping bags full of supplements they are giving their animals," says Donna Starita Mehan, DVM, of Boring, Oregon. "After a while the client becomes confused because the cat may not be making progress. I will do a muscle test on an animal with these supplements and sometimes find that one or two products will do the job and the others are unnecessary, an overkill that may even be hampering progress. This is where the individualized treatment that a holistic veterinarian can offer is invaluable in fine-tuning the needs of a particular cat."

It's important to remember that supplements are supplements. They are not meant to replace good food. Improve the diet first, then add the proper supplements. Until you have advice from a professional for your cat's particular condition, here are some general supplement recommendations that can apply to a broad spectrum of animals:

- **Multivitamins.** This is your basic supplement. A product with a wide array of nutrients fortifies the diet and compensates for possible deficiencies in food. In recent years an increasing number of excellent supplements have been formulated for pets and are available in health food and pet stores or through veterinarians.

- **Calcium.** Be cautious. Oversupplementing can cause problems, including urinary disorders, as cats get older. "The rule of thumb is to supplement if you are feeding homemade meals and not to add calcium if you are using strictly a commercial food," says Nancy Scanlan, DVM. She recommends 50 to 100 milligrams daily. Increase the amount by 25 percent for kittens.

- **Digestive enzymes.** Holistic veterinarians frequently recommend plant-based enzymes to optimize digestion, even for healthy cats, and routinely prescribe them for patients with digestive disorders. These products also aid older animals with slowing or diminished enzyme production. Special enzymes for pets are widely available.

- **Essential fatty acids.** Veterinarians frequently prescribe these supplements to improve the skin and combat exterior problems. There are many fatty acid products for pets on the market. If your animal is prone to inflammatory conditions such as chronic skin problems, use flaxseed oil, which is high in beneficial fatty acids. Start with perhaps 1 drop and gradually increase to a level equivalent to 1 teaspoon per fifteen pounds of body weight. You will find the flaxseed oil in the refrigeration section of a health food store. Look for organic products in dark containers, as this oil is quite fragile and will break down when exposed to light and heat. Buy a small bottle. Use it up and then buy another small bottle. That way the oil you serve is likely to be fresh.

- **Taurine.** This amino acid has been a thorny issue for years. Cats must obtain the nutrient in their diets. In the wilds the raw prey that cats historically have lived on supplied adequate taurine. With the advent of commercial pet food, cats began developing specific problems that were eventually traced to a taurine deficiency in the diet. The problems included blindness from retinal degeneration, reproductive defects, and dilated cardiomyopathy, a disease leading to heart failure. After

researchers discovered the taurine connection, pet food manufacturers added this critical nutrient to their formulations.
Nevertheless, some taurine-related problems have persisted
even when cats are fed fortified commercial foods. Taurine is
found in muscle meat, and a diet high in fresh, raw meat
should satisfy a cat's need. Meat processing and handling may
cause some loss of the nutrient. Beef is a poorer source of taurine than other meats. With all the uncertainties regarding this
critical nutrient, and as insurance against potential problems,
it's a good idea to supplement a cat with 60 to 80 milligrams of
taurine daily for each ten pounds of body weight.

- **Vitamin C.** 250 milligrams a day is recommended for general
  maintenance.

- **Vitamin E.** 50 international units (IU) a day. This nutrient is
  particularly useful for older cats.

HOW TO GIVE SUPPLEMENTS TO YOUR CAT

Supplements come in powder, capsule, and tablet form. Powders are
mixed directly in the food. You can pill a cat with a tablet or capsule,
but you will probably find it easier to empty the contents of capsules
into the food and do the same with crunched-up tablets. It is always
a good idea to start with a small amount and then work up slowly to
the suggested level. Start low. Go slow. This gives the cat a chance
to become accustomed to a new smell or taste. Administering supplements or any remedy or medicine to a cat can be a major challenge. For practical ideas on how to overcome resistance, see tips for
dosing cats at the beginning of part 2.

HOW TO FIND
A NUTRITIONALLY ORIENTED VETERINARIAN

Contact the American Holistic Veterinary Medical Association,
2214 Old Emmorton Rd., Bel Air, MD 21015 (phone: 410-
569-0795). If you have Internet access, use the directory of veterinarians on the alternative veterinary medicine Web site at
www.altvetmed.com.

8

Herbs

HERBS ARE FOOD for health. Carnivores like cats evolved not just on the meat they devour, but also on the greens present in the digestive tracts of their plant-eating prey. Even house cats will instinctively search out and chew plants and grass for ingredients missing in their diets. Such ingredients include vitamins, minerals, chlorophyll, and enzymes—whole-food factors necessary for health.

Herbs have been used since time immemorial by humans for healing purposes. All over the world native herbalists developed vast repertoires based on plants growing in their regions. They recognized specific medicinal properties contained in the roots, stems, seeds, flowers, bark, and leaves. These properties create a variety of known effects in the body, such as soothing, relaxing, lubricating, detoxifying, liquifying, stimulating, tonifying, and absorbing.

In recent years medical research and clinical usage of herbs have soared as modern science validates many of the traditional applications and explores new ones. Today herbal supplements are riding high atop a huge consumer wave of interest in natural healing.

Experts say the natural compounds in herbs—called "phytochemicals"—may offer the best protection against the diseases that plague society. There is much yet to learn about the tissue-specific way these compounds work. But in time they are expected to play a major role in antiaging medicine and how we prevent and treat disease.

HOW TO GIVE HERBS TO YOUR CAT

- Use whichever form of a recommended herb is easiest for you to administer. Herbs come as tablets, capsules, and liquid tinctures.

- Herbs are best given apart from a meal. Most are absorbed better this way. However, medicinal herbs often have a bitter or unpleasant taste. It is okay to mix them into food if that is the only way your cat will take them. Remember that taste is supreme for cats. So you will have to sneak the herb in slowly with a food the cat likes. For additional tips on giving supplements and remedies to very fussy cats, refer to the introduction to part 2.

- Chinese herbals come in tablet or pill form and do not taste good. Unless you can give pills to your cat, Chinese herbal formulas can be difficult to administer.

- Some tinctures have a strong odor that will repel cats. You can overcome that obstacle by putting the recommended amount in a capsule and pilling the cat, or diluting the tincture in a small quantity of a highly aromatic substance, such as tuna oil, and mixing it into the food.

- Some herbs have the potential to cause slight nausea. If there are signs of that, or an animal loses appetite when on herbs, administer on a full stomach.

- Unless you are knowledgeable about herbs, be careful when mixing them. Stick to tried-and-true formulas.

- Don't use willow bark for cats. This traditional herb often used for pain has the potential to be toxic to felines and cause ulcers.

HERBAL DOSAGES

In part 2 you will find many herbal recommendations for specific conditions. Included are herbs from Chinese medicine, from the Ayurvedic tradition of India, and from North and South America. The information will guide you on dosage and also on how to obtain a particular herbal product. Be sure to follow the instructions. In the current boom of interest in holistic health, people are jumping on the herbal bandwagon. However, it pays to be cautious when giving herbs to pets. Even though herbs are natural and can do much good, there is still potential for harm if they are given inappropriately or excessively.

There are no precise doses for pets. Veterinarians generally extrapolate their dosages according to the size of the animal. For cats they often use about one-eighth of the amount in tablet or capsule form recommended for people. For herbal tinctures they suggest using only a few drops twice a day. These are general recommendations. For specific herbs that are recommended in part 2 of this book, please follow the dosage advice for the individual herb.

Unless otherwise directed by a veterinarian, it is a good idea to start with a very small amount and work up slowly so as to avoid rejection and the possibility of stomach upset. Many times a low dose is enough and you don't have to go higher. An animal will resonate with the frequency of the herb, or the herb just isn't giving the animal what it needs. Giving more doesn't necessarily give more effect. Herbs heal by frequency, not necessarily by quantity.

THE "HEALING CRISIS"—MARK HAVERKOS, DVM

Herbs are capable of creating powerful healing effects in the body and may trigger a "healing crisis." This term, used by holistic healers, refers to a wave of purification generated by the natural medicine. Unlike conventional drugs, which suppress symptoms, herbs activate and fortify the body, like recharging a battery, helping it to cleanse itself of toxins and pathogens. In this process symptoms may temporarily intensify as a result. Things may get worse before they get better. It is then advisable to back off from the herb and let the body do the job it has now been activated to do. Improvement usually follows. You can then resume the remedy at the same or lesser level, depending on the situation. However, if the animal doesn't get better when the remedy is stopped, you should seek professional advice, preferably with a holistic veterinarian familiar with herbs.

HOW TO FIND A VETERINARIAN WHO USES HERBS

Contact the American Holistic Veterinary Medical Association, 2214 Old Emmorton Rd., Bel Air, MD 21015 (phone: 410-569-0795). If you have Internet access, use the directory of veterinarians on the alternative veterinary medicine Web site at www.altvetmed.com.

9

Homeopathic Remedies

HOMEOPATHY HAS LONG been popular in Europe and Asia, where kings, queens, and commoners alike have confidently relied on homeopathic remedies for their health needs. In North America the practice is rapidly gaining adherents among health-conscious consumers, and today homeopathy is a fast-growing part of the natural healing movement. It offers safe and effective treatments for many people problems, and for pet problems as well.

Among the most avid enthusiasts are members of the British royal family. Queen Elizabeth never travels without taking a kit of homeopathic medicines with her. Her thoroughbred horses and Welsh Corgi dogs are routinely treated homeopathically.

In France, a hotbed of homeopathy, some 1,000 veterinarians use it exclusively in the treatment of both large and small animals. The American Holistic Veterinary Medical Association includes more than 250 veterinarians who specialize in homeopathy or who use it along with other treatment techniques. The veterinarians say that just about every condition encountered in a general practice—from trauma to chronic disease—can be treated wholly or in part with homeopathy. Often the animals they see have undergone conventional treatment that hasn't worked or has caused too many side effects. Homeopathy offers a safe alternative. It is also an excellent complement to surgery and is frequently used to reduce postsurgical pain and accelerate the healing process.

Ideally, homeopathic veterinarians like to see animals treated homeopathically from early on. "Pets cared for this way live long, healthy lives and do not develop as many nagging health problems or serious illnesses," says Christina Chambreau, DVM. "At the ends of their lives, these animals tend to die from very short-term illnesses. As far as treating disease is concerned, homeopathy doesn't just relieve symptoms. It can restore health!"

As an example, Chambreau cites the case of a domestic shorthair cat who had been licking its belly raw for eight of its nine years. It had been receiving steroid shots from another veterinarian every six weeks and had many other lesser problems. After homeopathic treatment of about nine months and switching to a raw food diet, the cat stopped licking its belly. The animal lived to be seventeen and was sick only twice. It had a glowing hair coat until its death, which came suddenly from a kidney problem that lasted one week. "This is typical of animals who are maintained homeopathically," she says.

In part 2 of this book you will find many recommendations for homeopathic remedies. These natural medicines are available at health food stores, pharmacies, and holistic pet stores.

HOW HOMEOPATHIC REMEDIES WORK

Homeopathy utilizes remedies made from diluted amounts of natural substances—such as herbs, bark, seeds, berries, minerals, and animal matter. The remedies activate the body's own healing mechanisms according to a principle known as "like cures like." Here's how the principle works: These natural substances, given in large doses to healthy individuals or animals, will produce the same symptoms that they help heal when given in diluted homeopathic doses. It's simple yet hard to believe.

Two examples will help illustrate the point. A large amount of coffee can cause nervousness and prevent sleep. In homeopathy a remedy made from coffee is used to calm the nerves and help promote sleep. Sulfur, in a large dose, can cause a rash. In homeopathic amounts it helps heal rashes and skin problems and is a popular remedy for those conditions in animals.

Homeopathic remedies are so diluted that there is virtually no trace of the original substance. For this reason they are not toxic. Homeopathy works as an "energy medicine." The healing power comes not from the substances themselves, but from matching the energy vibration of a specific remedy to the energy pattern of the patient.

"Homeopathic remedies provide information to the body," says John Limehouse, DVM, of North Hollywood, California. "Imagine those card keys that open your hotel room. The right information on that magnetic strip will open the door. Similarly, homeopathic remedies contain magnetic resonance information. The right remedy contains the right information to stimulate the body's vital forces to do the work of healing, repair, and maintenance in a more efficient way."

How do homeopathic medicines compare to pharmaceutical drugs? Powerful medications often suppress symptoms and potentially lower the health status of the body by driving the disease deeper. Instead of suppressing symptoms, the correctly prescribed homeopathic remedy will safely, gently, and permanently elevate the health of the body.

WHAT A HOMEOPATHIC VETERINARIAN DOES

Hyperthyroidism, an overly active thyroid gland, has become common among cats. The signs are excessive appetite, weight loss, vomiting, and skin problems. This is a difficult disease to treat because it is a very deep condition. When it manifests, conventional medicine does one of three things: 1) surgical removal of the gland; 2) radioactive iodine treatment; or 3) Tapazol, a drug that reduces the function of the thyroid. All three situations have substantial drawbacks.

The homeopathic approach is to treat the whole animal and not just a single symptom or disease. Homeopathic practitioners prescribe specific remedies based on a variety of details, such as the color of a discharge, an animal's behavior and need for companionship or solitude, how it reacts to pain, when the pain is worse, and other factors that aggravate an illness. When they treat a hyperthyroid cat, the symptoms improve, and in the long run the thyroid function frequently normalizes.

"We seek clues to give us the right homeopathic remedy," explains Charles Loops, DVM, of Pittsboro, North Carolina. "If you select the correct remedy, then not only do the symptoms of pain and inflammation go away in the case of arthritis, for instance, but the animal is likely to be more energetic and feel better overall. Usually, if there is not a lot of tissue damage, you need give the remedy only for a short period of time and then go months or even years without having to use it again. Compare this to a drug that you have to use continually, running the risk of side effects and negative changes to the physiology. Basically, with homeopathy there are no side effects, only side benefits."

Homeopathic veterinarians typically prescribe a remedy or series of remedies with a single ingredient. Over-the-counter homeopathic remedies include single remedies as well as user-friendly combination formulas for people with little knowledge of homeopathy. Combinations include products for pets that have multiple ingredients to cover such problems as flea-bite allergic reactions, scratching, stress, motion sickness, and diarrhea. If you find that a combination does not help, it should be discontinued and the right single remedy found.

To effectively deal homeopathically with serious disorders, it is advisable to consult with a knowledgeable veterinarian. That's because it often takes skilled detective work to sort out the clues and select correct remedies. Moreover, many conditions are commonly aggravated by multiple, confusing factors, such as poor nutrition, vaccinations, and conventional drugs. Expertise is often needed to prescribe different remedies or potencies for changing conditions and symptoms.

Homeopathic specialists emphasize the importance of good nutrition and say that true healing is difficult without it, no matter how many remedies they prescribe. Some degree of illness is always going to be present unless an animal has a good nutritional basis.

Homeopaths also advise that it is best not to resort to "quick fix" pharmaceutical treatments of a symptom while using a homeopathic remedy because you will not know if an animal is improving or not.

UNDERSTANDING HOMEOPATHIC POTENCIES

Homeopathic remedies are identified by a name and number, such as Arnica 6X or 30C. The number tells you the potency—that is, the strength—of the particular remedy.

Remedies are created by a special process of consecutive dilutions in distilled water followed by succussion (vigorous shaking). X potencies refer to substances diluted 1 part to 9 parts of water. The designation 6X means the remedy was diluted and shaken 6 times. C potencies mean a substance has been diluted 1 part to 99 parts water. Thus 30C means a remedy that underwent 30 rounds of dilution and shaking.

This process is called "potentization." The more a substance is potentized—that is, diluted and shaken—the longer and more deeply the remedy acts in the body and the fewer doses are required for treatment.

Stores generally carry potencies of 30C or less. Higher potencies should be used cautiously, and ideally under the guidance of a professional. That's because higher potencies are more likely to trigger what is called a "healing crisis," in which symptoms may at first appear aggravated before they improve.

HOW TO GIVE HOMEOPATHIC REMEDIES TO YOUR CAT

Remedies come in several forms—liquid, pellets, and hard and soft tablets. There is no difference in effectiveness.

To give liquid remedies: Pull the lower cheek away from your cat's teeth. Using the dropper from the bottle, apply drops into the space between the gums and teeth. Do not touch the dropper to the skin or gum tissue. If you do, wash it afterward with boiling water before reusing. Liquid remedies contain a small amount of alcohol, which veterinary homeopaths say is not a problem, even for smaller animals. Occasionally the alcohol may cause a cat to foam at the mouth. If this happens, dilute the remedy until there is no foaming. Because this is an energy medicine, such dilution does not alter the effectiveness.

To give pellets and hard tablets: Spill out the pellets or tablets from the container onto a piece of white paper or an index card. Fold the paper repeatedly and then crush the remedy with the back of a spoon or a glass. Then sprinkle the powder into the front of your cat's mouth or into the space between the gums and teeth.

To give soft tablets: The soft tablets dissolve readily and do not need to be crushed. Simply place in the mouth.

HOMEOPATHIC DOSAGES

The quantity of the homeopathic remedy you administer is the same regardless of the size of your cat. Give enough so that you are sure some of the remedy goes into the mouth and is absorbed. Depending on the form of the remedy you use, a general rule of thumb is several tablets, or 3 to 5 tiny pellets, or a half dropperful of liquid.

When giving remedies on a regular basis, continually evaluate how your cat is doing. Keep a record of symptoms. If most symptoms become worse, or your cat is not feeling happier and more active, then the remedies aren't working. This is the time to consult with an experienced homeopath.

A onetime single dose should always be administered directly into the mouth. For repeated doses, the remedy can be added to, or dissolved in drinking water if it is not easy to give by mouth. If the cat doesn't drink much water, but likes cream or milk, the remedy can be dissolved in those liquids. It is best, especially for single doses, not to give the remedy within an hour before or after feeding.

Unless you are being guided by a specialist, don't give the same remedy on a daily basis for more than about two weeks. Constant administration of a remedy can create the symptoms or toxic effects you are attempting to counteract.

FOR MORE INFORMATION ON HOMEOPATHY

- *The Consumer's Guide to Homeopathy*, by Dana Ullman (Tarcher-Putnam), an excellent introduction to homeopathic healing. For this and other books, contact Ullman's Homeopathic Educational Services, 2124 Kittredge St., Berkeley, CA 94704 (phone: 510-649-0294).

- The following books from England, also available through the Homeopathic Educational Services, offer specific information about homeopathy and companion animals:
    The Homeopathic Treatment of Small Animals by Christopher Day.
    Cats: Homeopathic Remedies by George MacLeod.
    The Treatment of Cats by Homeopathy by K. Sheppard.

- Write to Christina Chambreau, DVM, 908 Cold Bottom Rd., Sparks, MD, 21152, for information on homeopathy seminars for pet owners.

HOW TO FIND A VETERINARY HOMEOPATH

Contact the Academy of Veterinary Homeopathy, at 751 N.E. 168th St., N. Miami, FL 33162-2427 (phone: 305-652-1590).

Contact the American Holistic Veterinary Medical Association, 2214 Old Emmorton Rd., Bel Air, MD 21015 (phone: 410-569-0795). If you have Internet access, use the directory of veterinarians on the alternative veterinary medicine Web site at www.altvetmed.com.

⩕ 10 ⩕

Flower Essences—Healing the Emotions

IF YOU BELIEVE in the mind-body connection, you're going to love flower essences. This unique healing system was developed by an English physician, Edward Bach. During the 1930s he discovered that many of the nonpoisonous wild plants, bushes, and trees in the English countryside exerted genuine therapeutic effects on the emotions, which in turn promoted physical balance in the body. He believed that by thus correcting emotional dysfunction, you could help heal physical dysfunction.

Bach identified and developed applications for thirty-eight individual English flower essences plus the well-known five-flower combination called Rescue Remedy. Since his time, many more flower essences have been added. Today there is even a whole new breed of products called "nature essences" that work on the same principle and are prepared from gems, minerals, and animal matter. The original essences, as well as the newer additions, are available at most health food stores and come in a liquid form.

Each individual remedy relates to a specific mental and emotional state. Bach once declared that disease is a kind of consolidation of a mental attitude...and that behind all disease lie our fears, our anxieties, our greed, and our likes and dislikes.

Flower remedies have been most widely used for humans, where stressful and negative emotional states are known to weaken the immune system and contribute to the disease process. Veterinarians, too, have been using and prescribing these essences for many years and in increasing numbers find them highly beneficial to help heal the emotional and physical ills of dogs and cats.

Jean Hofve, DVM, has extensively studied and used flower essences for many species of animals. "They often bring remarkable results in cats, dogs, horses, and wildlife," she says. "We know that in humans, mental and emotional upset can have deep and lasting physical effects, far beyond what used to be referred to as 'psychosomatic illness.' Animals, too, have an active mental and emotional life. They can similarly manifest not only behavioral but physical problems that have their roots in emotional trauma."

Writing in *Complementary and Alternative Veterinary Medicine* (Mosby, St. Louis, 1998), Stephen Blake, DVM, points out that he has used flower remedies effectively for more than ten years. "Most pet owners and veterinarians would agree that behavioral problems are a major concern," says Blake. "They often accompany or precede physical disease as well. The dramatic positive changes in the animals' behavior demonstrates the effectiveness of the noninvasive way the remedies work…[to] alleviate the emotional stresses in veterinary patients."

HOW FLOWER ESSENCES WORK

Flower essences basically correct a negative emotional state by "flooding" the patient with the opposite, positive quality that is the particular essence of that flower. For instance, the essence of the flower Holly is love. Therefore you would use Holly in situations where there is a lack of love, as in times of jealousy, anger, or hatred. Rock Rose, another essence, holds the quality of courage and is used in times of deep fears, panic, and terror.

With flower remedies you aren't treating specific behavior. You are working on a subtle emotional level instead, trying to create a new mental state that is peaceful and happy. Hofve says that while flower essences can be used for physical conditions, she believes their greatest application is to help correct behavioral problems, many of which are based on emotional or mental disturbances. She has found that these remedies work between 70 and 100 percent of the time.

Flower remedies are generally considered an "energy medicine," as are homeopathic remedies. Essences, however, are not prepared in the same way as homeopathics. Part of the essence processing, for instance, involves infusion of the liquid extract with sunlight.

Experts say flower remedies enhance the effectiveness of any form of medicine, conventional or alternative, without any interference. They cannot be overused or misused, and if you administer the wrong remedy, it will simply not have any effect. Essences are safe and nontoxic.

In part 2 of this book you will find a number of flower essence recommendations from veterinarians for behavioral problems. If you do not have a successful result, seek out a veterinarian knowledgeable in the method.

HOW TO GIVE LIQUID FLOWER ESSENCES TO YOUR CAT

1. **By mouth.** The liquid doesn't need to be swallowed. It is enough just for the liquid to contact the mucous membranes of the gums or tongue. Try not to contaminate the dropper by touching it to the animal. In case this occurs, rinse the dropper in boiling water before returning it to the bottle.

2. **Applied topically,** usually around the head and ears. You can even put a few drops in your hand and pat your cat on the head.

3. **Added to an animal's wet food or water.** There is no loss of potency from dilution.

4. **Add a dropperful to a spray bottle filled with spring water.** Spray rooms, carriers, cars, houses, trailers, or stalls.

FLOWER ESSENCE DOSAGES

Generally, give 4 to 8 drops at a time. For most behavioral problems, give three to four times a day for two to four weeks. If the response is adequate by then, decrease the frequency.

In crisis situations, such as the loss of a loved one, a tornado, or some sudden fearful event, the remedy can be given as often as needed, even every few minutes. For chronic behavioral problems, such as cats not getting along well, you may need to add a dropperful to the drinking water or give directly one or more times a day long-term. The speed of response generally depends on the condition and how long it has been present. Usually you should notice a change within two weeks.

FOR MORE INFORMATION ON FLOWER ESSENCES

- Additional remedy options and instructions on how to mix your own combinations are found in an Internet article by Hofve at the Critter Chat on-line newsletter at www.critterhaven.org/critterchat/bach.htm, or visit her Web site at www.spiritessence.com.

- Flower Essence Society, P.O. Box 459, Nevada City, CA 95959. Phone: 800-736-9222 or 530-265-9163. Web site: www.flowersociety.org.

- Nelson Bach USA, 100 Research Dr., Wilmington, MA 01887. Phone: 978-988-3833 for information; 800-314-BACH for orders. Web site: www.bachcentre.com.

HOW TO FIND A VETERINARIAN
USING FLOWER ESSENCES

Contact the American Holistic Veterinary Medical Association, 2214 Old Emmorton Rd., Bel Air, MD 21015 (phone: 410-569-0795). If you have Internet access, use the directory of veterinarians on the alternative veterinary medicine Web site at www.altvetmed.com.

11

Veterinary Acupuncture

THE ANCIENT CHINESE practice of acupuncture, which has gained major recognition in mainstream Western medicine, is not just for people. It works superbly for pain and for acute and chronic disorders in pets and is also a first-class tool for preventive health care. Acupuncture is not anything you can do on your own. You need to bring your animal to a specialist. It's well worth the money. Acupuncture generates powerful and often amazing relief and curative benefits, as either a primary treatment or in support of standard procedures, for numerous problems that are difficult to treat conventionally.

WHAT IS ACUPUNCTURE?

Acupuncture is based on the Chinese healing principle of *qi* (pronounced "chee"), which loosely means "energy," and its effect on body functions. During an acupuncture treatment, needles, with or without microelectrical currents attached, are inserted at specific bodily locations along meridians of energy. The needles stimulate sensory nerve endings that send impulses up through the spinal cord to the different areas of the brain, causing both local- and central-acting effects. By stimulating these points, acupuncturists seek to unblock energy "bottlenecks" and restore normal energy flow. The process stimulates the body's ability to heal itself. On the local level, the technique relieves muscle spasm and increases circulation. Systemically it causes release of different neurotransmitters and hormones throughout the body.

Veterinarians trained in acupuncture say their technique puts an animal's energy back in balance whether they are treating a kidney, liver, pancreas, or arthritic condition.

DO THE NEEDLES HURT?

What about cats being stuck with needles? Will they sit for it? Is it painful? Pet owners always ask those questions before their animal receives a first treatment. Well, the experts say you can relax, because animals normally don't mind it, and, in fact, many cats seem to enjoy it.

When an acupuncture needle is inserted, it pushes tissue out of the way, causing very little, if any, discomfort. This is due in part to specially designed fine wire needles that have no edges. They literally slip into holes that lead to the actual acupuncture point.

Nancy Scanlan, DVM, has found that cats actually "love" the treatment. "I find cats are very responsive, more so than dogs, and because of this I can use fewer needles than for a dog," she says. "The first time they may be a little uptight. But after one or two treatments they often will come right out of their carrier—which they never do at an animal hospital—and curl right up against me ready for another treatment. Anyone who doesn't believe in acupuncture should just observe a cat before and after treatment. Older cats have a lot of pain going on, and back problems, even though it may not show as arthritis on an X-ray. Many cats will stop jumping up on chairs or tables, and you may think the animal is getting weak. After acupuncture they usually start jumping back up again."

Veterinary acupuncturists say that when they encounter a fearful or overanxious cat, they are usually able to calm the animal and proceed with the treatment by using natural relaxants such as flower essences, homeopathics, or herbs. Occasionally a mild tranquilizer may be necessary.

HOW ACUPUNCTURE CAN HELP YOUR CAT

Acupuncturists find they frequently can enhance the quality of life— and even extend life—for cases where other veterinarians have nothing more to offer. Pamela Wood-Krzeminski, DVM, for instance, says she successfully uses a combination of acupuncture and Chinese herbs to help most of the chronic kidney patients referred to her who have reached the end of the line with conventional medicine.

Joseph Demers, DVM, uses the technique to effectively deal with serious feline urinary infections. "Most of these cases involve chronic infections, animals who have been on long-term antibiotics," he reports. "But with a few treatments of acupuncture, along with a good diet, we can achieve total remission in many cases or a significant reduction in the frequency of infections. When the infection recurs, a single acupuncture treatment generally resolves the problem."

Lynne Friday, DVM, of Lexington, Michigan, reports that acupuncture can help many cases of nongenetic hearing loss that often occurs in older animals. "I can usually restore about 50 percent of the hearing with four to ten treatments," she says.

Specialists say acupuncture can often eliminate the need for surgery.

Among the areas most responsive to acupuncture in cats are the following:

- **Pain relief.** Some veterinarians say it is the best pain reliever of all the alternative therapies, especially for chronic pain.

- **Musculoskeletal problems,** such as arthritis, lameness, and stiff backs in older cats. Experienced acupuncturists say they can effectively help more than three-quarters of the cases they treat.

- **Certain neurological problems,** such as epilepsy.

- **Gastrointestinal disorders** such as chronic vomiting, diarrhea, and constipation.

- **Immune system enhancement.** Acupuncture can be a useful adjunct in the treatment of feline leukemia and immunodeficiency virus.

- **Postponement of surgery in high risk cases.** Acupuncture can help patients gain strength.

• **Postsurgical promotion of healing.** After an operation, some animals will have lingering pain or discomfort at the site of surgery and start chewing or licking the spot. Acupuncture can often stop it. After surgery involving the legs, animals will sometimes have trouble walking. Acupuncture can help restore full motion.

HOW MANY TREATMENTS ARE CUSTOMARY?

An individual acupuncture session might last a few seconds or up to an hour. Your cat's condition and response determine the number and frequency of office visits required. In general, the longer a problem has existed, and the more serious it is, the greater the number of treatments necessary. Veterinarians say they have had severe cases that responded dramatically to one treatment, while other cases that seemed to be quite mild required several treatments. Sometimes the results of a single treatment are long-lasting. Other times a series of treatments is necessary for a long-lasting effect. No two cases are the same.

HOW TO FIND A VETERINARY ACUPUNCTURIST

Contact the International Veterinary Acupuncture Society, P.O. Box 1478, Longmont, CO 80502 (phone: 303-449-7936).

Contact the American Holistic Veterinary Medical Association, 2214 Old Emmorton Rd., Bel Air, MD 21015 (phone: 410-569-0795). If you have Internet access, use the directory of veterinarians on the alternative veterinary medicine Web site at www.altvetmed.com.

☙ 12 ☙

Veterinary Chiropractic

IN RECENT YEARS many holistic veterinarians have become trained in chiropractic methods and apply them therapeutically for a number of conditions, either as a primary or a supportive treatment.

Chiropractic involves a system of locating spinal and joint misalignments throughout the body and "adjusting" them through a series of treatments that reduce the stressful impact on the nervous system and organs. Such misalignments pinch nerves and cause pain as well as disturbances to normal behavioral and physical functioning. Misalignments commonly occur from injury, birth trauma, and wear and tear of the body. They can also result from malnutrition and toxicity, often present to some degree in chronic diseases. Thus, in many cases of prolonged illness, an undiagnosed misalignment may be present that is contributing to the problem.

Without chiropractic evaluation, such misalignments usually go undiagnosed and may produce a lifetime of suffering. The aim of chiropractic is to restore the normal structural alignment of the body so that energy flows better and moving parts work more optimally.

"I use chiropractic to get animals to feel better and give them more ease and flexibility," says Mark Haverkos, DVM. "When animals feel better, they function better. I often see immediate results after a single adjustment."

Veterinary chiropractors sometimes combine chiropractic with acupuncture. They use the acupuncture first to relax the muscles of an animal, enabling them to make more effective realignments.

HOW CHIROPRACTIC CAN HELP YOUR CAT

Most typically, veterinarians use chiropractic methods when treating cats for musculoskeletal problems stemming from arthritic changes and injury. Older cats often develop joint stiffness and problems in the spine, the result of a lifetime of minor trauma generated from jumping and running. These small injuries are not apparent at the time they occur, but they add up and may eventually slow an animal down.

Many cats suffer from subtle misalignments undetected by X-rays. Though subtle, they have the potential at any time in life to upset the normal biomechanics of motion and cause inflammation and degeneration of tissue. These situations are often resolved by gentle chiropractic adjustments. Lameness, for which the cause has not been found, is an example. Either the hips or the forelegs may be involved. Frequently the pet owner believes the cause is arthritis, yet X-rays are negative. The problem instead may stem from a nerve impingement from a spinal or joint misalignment that develops pain or reduces nerve supply to a leg, similar to sciatica in humans.

You may be surprised to know that veterinarians have considerable success treating many behavioral problems with chiropractic that do not respond to other treatments. The overlooked cause of the problem could be a structural misalignment in the neck or, even more overlooked, a misalignment of the skull bones.

Roger DeHaan, DVM, has found such misalignments in more than a third of the chronic behavioral cases he treats. "There is a jamming or pinching of the cranial plates, which can lead to headaches, irritability, hyperactivity, or depression," he says. "I have dramatic, and sometimes instant, success in many of these cases using chiropractic cranial adjustments." One outstanding case cited by DeHaan involved a cat who hadn't been eating. The owners had taken it to a prestigious clinic, where the animal was hospitalized for ten days. The specialists could find nothing wrong, and the cat was not responsive to medication. The owner then brought the cat to DeHaan, who determined the presence of misalignments in the skull that in some way were obstructing normal nerve impulses and affecting appetite. The veterinarian says that one treatment restored the cat's normal appetite.

The skull is not one solid piece of bone. Rather, it comprises plates that actually move, similar in a way to how the geological plates in the earth move. When you breathe in and out, for instance, the skull bones shift microscopically. Head or neck trauma can cause the bones to lock along the suture lines—the fault lines, so to speak—that separate the plates. Inadequate prenatal nutrition and difficult delivery can also cause misaligned cranial bones. Whatever the cause, the resultant loss of movement can create neurological disturbances, stress, abnormal function, and symptoms.

HOW MANY TREATMENTS ARE CUSTOMARY?

Ron Carsten, DVM, of Glenwood Springs, Colorado, recalls the case of a domestic shorthair cat suffering from lameness in a front leg for more than a year. Two other veterinarians had previously treated the animal with steroidal anti-inflammatories, but there was no response to the drugs. "I found a misalignment in the cervical [neck] spine," says Carsten. "One chiropractic adjustment eliminated the problem. It's been more than a year now, and the cat has had no recurrence of the lameness."

Dramatic success after one treatment, of course, doesn't happen in every case. The number of treatments depends on the condition. However, veterinary chiropractors say they are often able to restore normal alignment in situations like this with three or four sessions, sometimes even less.

HOW TO TELL IF YOUR CAT CAN BENEFIT
FROM CHIROPRACTIC TREATMENT

In general, if you encounter sensitivity when you stroke the backside, or when your cat isn't jumping up on the bed the way it used to, consider a chiropractic evaluation. Lynne Friday, DVM, has developed the following head-to-toe checklist of misalignment signs.

The neck may be misaligned if:
- The head is cocked to one side or the other.
- The cat is reluctant to raise the head or flex the neck without crying.

The jaw may be misaligned if:
- Kittens cry, become cranky, and appear uncomfortable when nursing.
- There is sudden behavioral change, particularly after the cat has undergone teeth cleaning or oral surgery or has been intubated.
- There is shaking of the head or scratching of the face or ear, especially on one side. This could also be a sign of cranial misalignment.
- Seizures occur where medication does not help.
- The mouth is sore when you try to open it.
- The cat has a distressed look or acts depressed. The head may be down. This could indicate a headache. If you are sensitive to your cat, you can tell there is pain by looking in the eyes.

The ribs, thoracic (upper back) vertebrae, or breastbone may be misaligned if:
- The cat walks almost on its tiptoes, as if walking on high heels. You can confirm this if you lift the animal with your hands under the chest and it cries out.

A spinal misalignment in the lower back may be involved if:
- The cat walks like a camel, with its back humped. This is called "splinting," an effort to hold itself together to take away pressure from the spinal cord as it stretches out. The cat is guarding the lower back.
- The cat cries when it sits and acts as if it is sitting on a cactus.

The pelvis or hip may be out of line if:
- The cat sits off to one side.

HOW TO FIND A VETERINARY CHIROPRACTOR

Contact the American Veterinary Chiropractic Association, 623 Main St., Hillsdale, IL 61257 (phone: 309-658-2920).

The American Holistic Veterinary Medical Association, 2214 Old Emmorton Rd. Bel Air, MD 21015 (phone: 410-569-0795). If you have Internet access, use the directory of veterinarians on the alternative veterinary medicine Web site at www.altvetmed.com.

⚊ 13 ⚊

Massage Techniques

THIS CHAPTER INTRODUCES four gentle hands-on techniques you can do on your own that generate healing energy and improve the physical health of your cat. The importance of human contact cannot be overemphasized. Petting and stroking keep you connected to your cat, creating an interchange of love and energy benefiting both you and your animal companion. Simple and gentle massages are a good way to take physical contact one step further, to a level of healing. If, through your massage activity, you detect a growth or area of extreme sensitivity or pain, be sure to bring it to your veterinarian's attention.

The Daily Health Massage—Norman Ralston, DVM
Start with gentle stroking of the ears in a circular, clockwise fashion. As you gently massage the ears, which are rich in acupuncture points, you are in a sense stimulating or treating every major organ in the body. You are sending a minute electrical impulse to each organ. Near the base of the ear is located the thermostat of the body. By massaging here, we also increase the temperature of the body. You can experience this by rubbing your own ears.

Once you have raised the energy by massaging the ears, gently stroke the cat from head to tail to direct the energy flow. Do this daily for a house pet if possible. Often when a problem is developing, a sensitivity will appear in an associated acupoint or meridian, sometimes twenty-four hours before symptoms show up. By understanding this and being aware that your cat has suddenly developed a sensitivity at a given point, you can, through gentle massage, cause the energy to flow to the part and stimulate healing before a major problem arises.

Massage for Back Pain and Stiffness—Nancy Scanlan, DVM

This light touch massage covers various acupuncture points on the body and acts in a sense as a very mild acupuncture treatment, releasing spasm and possible trigger points. For cats with pain and stiffness in the back, this massage generates more limberness.

Make small circles with two fingers of both hands, starting at the base of the ears, and slowly work your way down along both sides of the spine. Make two or three circles on the skin at each spot as you move down just to the right and the left of the spine, along the big muscles. Don't exert a lot of pressure and push on the muscles. Be delicate. Just move the skin over the muscles with a light touch. If you start massaging too hard, the muscles tense up, and the cat will want to get away, because it is painful.

Massage gently in this light touch manner down to the base of the tail and then back up again. If you hit a point where you notice an actual release of heat, that is an area of muscle spasm that has just relaxed. If you encounter this phenomenon, concentrate on the area. It will feel as if you have been on a heating pad at that spot.

Spinal Massages—Roger DeHaan, DVM

A gentle massage of the muscles along the spine helps work out tension and increase blood flow for cats with arthritis. It also serves as a general massage and puts energy into the body. The technique is simple and involves kneading or massaging the muscles in small clockwise circles.

To massage trouble spots along the spine, run the palm of your hand slowly just over the surface of the coat. Move your hand from the front to the rear, from the shoulder to the tailbone. Do this several times. Quietly notice if some areas give off an increase in heat. Any cat who has arthritis or trouble walking will give off more heat in certain spots. Those are areas of spasm or tension. You will be surprised how easy it is to feel the areas of heat. If you don't detect any heat, move your hand higher to about one to two inches above the body and again slowly move it from front to rear. Now you are attempting to detect "radiant heat" that may be emanating from the cat.

A second technique I call "the 4-4-4 rule" will help generate relief for any animal with mild back problems. Check with your veterinarian to be sure that there are no contraindications.

Hold the middle of the tail with your strong hand. Use the other hand for leverage, and hold on to the shoulder. Now *gently* tug on the tail for four seconds, as if it were a rope and you were pulling it away from the animal's body. Apply very mild pressure, the equivalent of pressing a bathroom scale to read one or two pounds. Then release the pressure for four seconds.

Do the maneuver a total of four times, increasing the traction *slightly* each time. Sometimes you will hear a pop, even in the tail, when a misalignment goes back into place. When doing this procedure, never apply too much pressure and never jerk the tail. If the animal doesn't like it, don't do it. Most like it, however.

All the vertebrae that run down the spine are connected, like a rope. This simple action opens microspaces along the length of the spine, allowing a bit more room for blood vessels and nerves that might otherwise be pinched.

Use this technique until the cat improves. I generally recommend it daily for a week, then two or three times for two weeks, and then as needed.

The Antianxiety Massage—Pamela Wood-Krzeminski, DVM

A simple method for calming anxiety or aggressive behavior is to massage an acupressure point on the head. If you have an acupuncture chart handy, it is point GV20. Specifically, it is located in the central indentation on the top of the skull that runs from front to back and just forward of a make-believe line connecting the ears. This is considered an energizing point for the front of the body.

Massage the point daily for thirty seconds to a minute in a clockwise direction. This has been shown in many cases to calm a nervous or aggressive cat. If you do this with an aggressive animal, just make sure you don't run the risk of getting bitten.

14

The Vaccination Question— How Often, How Much?

FOR YEARS HOLISTIC veterinarians have argued that standard vacci-nation procedures represent a medical overkill harming many pets. In their opinion, too many vaccines at one time and unnecessary annual revaccinations are the frequent cause of adverse reactions, weakened immune systems, and an assortment of chronic health problems.

Recently the veterinary profession has begun downshifting its recommendations for vaccinations and, most notably, the hallowed concept of annual boosters. A steady stream of evidence from lead-ing researchers has challenged the effectiveness and scientific valid-ity of the practice. Experts now say that almost without exception there is no immunological requirement for annual shots. Vaccina-tions enhance immunity against viruses and bacteria for years or perhaps even for the life of an animal. While defending the impor-tance that vaccines play in preventing, controlling, and eliminating fatal diseases in dogs and cats, prominent researchers say that the goal of the veterinary profession should be to vaccinate more ani-mals but vaccinate them less often and only with vaccines that are necessary for a particular animal.

Vaccination guidelines are in a state of transition. At the time of the writing of this book, the new thinking is that kittens should have an initial vaccination series for the most clinically important vac-cines, for which the duration of immunity is at least three years and probably more than five. Cats are routinely vaccinated for pan-leukopenia (cat distemper), upper-respiratory illnesses, and rabies. Vaccines are also available for feline leukemia, feline infectious peritonitis, and ringworm.

Holistic veterinarians welcome the changes as long overdue, steps in the right direction but still involving more vaccinations than most think are necessary. The emphasis of these professionals is on building up health through diet and natural healing, not on repeated vaccinations.

WHAT VETERINARIANS DON'T TELL YOU ABOUT VACCINATIONS

Holistic veterinarians disagree with mainstream veterinary organizations that downplay the risk and incidence of reactions to vaccinations. "Vaccinations help eradicate or reduce the incidence of severe, acute diseases, but the by-product has been to plague animals with insidious, chronic diseases that are very difficult to treat," says Charles Loops, DVM. "Vaccinations represent a major stress on the body, and especially when administered in the form of vaccine combinations that flood the body with millions of organisms or viral particles, causing turmoil in the immune system."

Reactions to vaccinations may be minor, such as fever, skin rashes, local irritations at the site of injections, and lack of appetite. However, many of the veterinarians interviewed for this book say they routinely treat cats, often brought to them as a last resort, who develop challenging health problems within days, weeks, or several months after vaccination. Some believe that repeated vaccinations even lay the groundwork for cancer. Common health problems cited as a consequence of vaccinations include the following:

- New or aggravated skin allergies or bowel disorders.
- Life-threatening autoimmune crises, where the body's immune system attacks healthy tissue, resulting in asthma, epilepsy, thyroid disease, and lupuslike symptoms.
- Undesirable behavior changes such as fearfulness and aggression.
- Weak animals going from bad to worse. Animals, unwell to begin with, now suffering from adrenal malfunction or even cancer.

- Animals who experience relapses when their owners allow them to be vaccinated during the course of holistic treatments.

Michele Yasson, DVM, of Rosendale, New York, regularly sees animals who have never been vaccinated and in old age are healthy and robust. "They seem to have a much lower incidence of chronic, debilitative, degenerative diseases such as diabetes, hypothyroidism, and cancer," she says. "Vaccines are like any disease influence—a harsh stimulus to the body. Some animals are more susceptible than others. I have some patients who have never been well since they were vaccinated."

THE PROMISE OF ANTIBODY TESTS

Among the new developments talked about by veterinarians are antibody titer tests, seen as a promising way to assess the need for additional vaccinations. Such tests determine the strength of an animal's immune system against a particular disease. "Practically speaking, cats should have antibody titers evaluated annually until we know how long the vaccination-induced antibodies actually last in the blood," says Susan Wynn, DVM, of Marietta, Georgia. "These annual tests will provide some peace of mind, while at the same time helping to establish just how long vaccinations actually protect the average animal. This is critical knowledge that will guide us how to more safely and judiciously vaccinate our pets and at the same time save many pets the ordeal of iatrogenic illnesses."

Nevertheless, these tests are not universally agreed upon as accurate and foolproof assessments of immune status. Low levels, as well as adequate levels, guarantee nothing, Wynn cautions, "just as simply giving a vaccination guarantees nothing in terms of an animal's immune response."

WHAT TO DO ABOUT VACCINATIONS

The definitive scientific verdict on the frequency and effectiveness of vaccinations lies in the future. Among veterinarians, opinions differ widely. Some holistic veterinarians, for instance, believe in not vaccinating at all, except for what the law demands (usually rabies shots). Others say to vaccinate kittens and then boost them at a year and then perhaps every five years. There is no consensus.

Your decision on vaccinations requires consideration of many factors:

- Are you committed to a nutritious diet that will optimize your cat's health?

- Is your cat healthy? Veterinarians say you should not vaccinate unhealthy animals.

- Unless absolutely necessary, you probably shouldn't vaccinate a cat with a history of reactions to vaccines. If vaccination is necessary, consult the guidelines in this chapter for preventing reactions.

- What is the potential for exposure to contagious microorganisms? Do you have an indoor animal, the only cat in the house? An outdoor prowler? Part of a multicat household or a cattery?

- In some states and municipalities, rabies vaccines are required by law. Check with your animal control authority for local regulations and for traveling out of state.

It is best to consult with your veterinarian, who should be aware of the latest thinking on vaccinations. If he or she isn't up-to-date, and simply recommends annual booster shots, you need another veterinarian. Ideally see a holistic veterinarian who can help you maximize the health of your pet and minimize the number of vaccinations.

In the meantime, consider the following general suggestions made by veterinarians interviewed for this book:

- Vaccinate only healthy animals. Weak animals often go from bad to worse.

- Split up vaccinations and do fewer at one time. It takes about twenty-one days for the immune system to complete its response to a vaccine. So wait at least three weeks, and preferably four, between vaccinations.

- Always ask for killed-cell vaccines, which are less expensive and have fewer potential side effects than modified-live vaccines. Donna Starita Mehan, DVM, believes that many of the chronic eye, bladder, upper-respiratory, and gum and mouth inflammatory conditions she treats are related to the modified-live herpes rhinotracheitis vaccine that animals have been receiving yearly. To test this connection, Mehan conducted an informal study among a litter of kittens in her Oregon clinic. One-half of the litter received live-virus vaccines, and all developed some form of chronic gingivitis or stomatitis, an inflammatory condition of the mucous membranes of the mouth. The kittens who received killed-cell vaccines had no problems. "This was by no means a controlled study, but the results along with many other observations over the years have led me to have little doubt that the live vaccines are causing stomatitis, upper-respiratory and bladder infections, and eye ulcers," says Mehan.

- Watch for any growths at the site of a vaccination injection. A harmless swelling frequently occurs at the site and usually disappears after several weeks. However, a tumor called a fibrosarcoma has been found occasionally to develop exactly where animals are vaccinated. Veterinarians should document where a shot is given, and owners should pay attention to the location as well. A higher than expected incidence of tumors has prompted some experts to even recommend injecting the hind leg to facilitate amputation if a tumor occurs. This is not a tumor that spreads throughout the body, but it is locally aggressive and invasive, and it tends to recur. If you notice any growth at the site, consult with your veterinarian.

- Animals with genetically based hormonal-immune imbalances may not develop protective antibodies from vaccinations. There are many such animals. Vaccines may be worthless for them. See the next chapter on immune-endocrine testing of hormonal-immune integrity and as an important indicator of whether vaccinations will "take" or not.

- Geriatric animals don't need shots. Most of the diseases vaccinated for affect younger animals.

REMEDIES FOR PREVENTING AND RELIEVING REACTIONS TO VACCINATIONS

Thuja is the leading homeopathic remedy to deal with vaccinosis—that is, adverse reactions to vaccinations. Consider it both preventively or if a problem develops after vaccination.

Dosage
- **Thuja 30C:** One dose within twenty-four hours of vaccination to prevent adverse reactions for cats with a history of post-vaccination problems. If a reaction occurs, give once a day for five days. Veterinarians say that cats with a history of vaccine reactions shouldn't be revaccinated unless it is absolutely necessary.

For cats who develop more severe vaccine reactions, Karen Bentley, DVM, recommends a combination homeopathic remedy called Vaccine Detox Tabs, by Natramed. It contains Thuja, Sulfur, Arsenicum album, Pulsatilla, Silicea, and Antimonium. The formula was developed by Asa Hershoff, N.D., a Southern California homeopathic physician. The product can be ordered in the United States, through Dr. Hershoff's Santa Monica office (310-829-7122); or in Canada, through Actiform in Markham, Ontario (800-668-0066).

Dosage
- Vaccine Detox Tabs 1 or 2 tablets daily, starting a week before vaccination. Finish the entire bottle. To remedy ongoing chronic problems resulting from past vaccines, give 1 tablet up to three times daily for two weeks or more.

ALTERNATIVES TO VACCINES—NOSODES

When pet owners ask about alternatives to vaccines, one possibility is a nosode, a homeopathic remedy prepared from an isolate of the particular disease agent. However, properly controlled studies have yet to be conducted on the effectiveness of this method, according to *Complementary and Alternative Veterinary Medicine*, the major reference book on holistic practices.

Among holistic veterinarians, opinion is divided. Some recommend them and say they have had good results. Others do not recommend them. If you are considering nosodes, consult with a holistic veterinarian who is familiar with them.

15

What to Do When Nothing Seems to Work

IF NOTHING SEEMS to work that you and your veterinarian try in order to improve your cat's health, consider the two unique tests—developed by veterinarians—described in this chapter. Both are available through your vet and can reveal critical clues for developing powerful hormonal and nutritional therapies. The tests can also be used to determine deficiencies and imbalances before problems occur so that an effective preventive strategy can be worked out.

TEST #1: THE ENDOCRINE-IMMUNE TEST
FOR GENETIC PROBLEMS

Sitting atop each kidney is the tiny, thumbnail-shaped adrenal gland, part of an exquisite network of glands called the endocrine system. The role of glands is to produce minute quantities of hormones, chemical substances with powerful regulating effects on the body's operation. The adrenals pump out a staggering array of important hormones, including estrogen, adrenaline, and cortisol. Cortisol regulates the activity of the white blood cells known as lymphocytes, immune cells that produce antibodies to counteract viruses, bacteria, disease, and toxic substances. Cortisol, in turn, is regulated by a hormone produced by the pituitary gland. This hormone controls cortisol production depending on whether there is too much or too little cortisol circulating in the body.

The pituitary-adrenal relationship is just one of many finely tuned feedback mechanisms within the endocrine system that governs a major branch of the body's defense forces. When the system is operating smoothly, the white blood cells naturally recognize the difference between friend and foe. They turn their chemical weapons on the enemy. They do not attack healthy tissue. The hand of man, however, has overturned this remarkable arrangement in many of our cats.

"Years of inbreeding and line breeding in a one-pointed attempt to achieve certain cosmetic appearances for sales or show ribbons have upset the precision of these systems and perpetuated the breeding of genetically flawed animals, contributing in a big way to today's epidemic of disease among companion animals," says Alfred Plechner, DVM.

The Los Angeles veterinarian, who has investigated this issue for more than twenty years, believes that the critical regulating mechanisms linking the endocrine and the immune system have been seriously damaged. Many animals can't produce enough cortisol, or what they do produce is inactive. Their other hormones are out of balance as well. The flaws are passed down from generation to generation, from purebreds to purebreds, from purebreds to mixed breeds, and from mixed breeds to other mixed breeds.

COMMON TYPES OF ENDOCRINE-IMMUNE DISORDERS

The end result is the proliferation of cats programmed for self-destruction, says Plechner. Their internal systems are out of control. They have all the medical diseases that the veterinary profession has trouble treating:

- Severe hypersensitivity.
- Relentless skin allergies with inflammation, ulceration, and itchiness.
- Chronic vomiting and diarrhea.
- Generalized mange.
- Aggressiveness, rage, and weird behavior. Male and female cats both spraying walls, chasing owners, and defecating in improper places.
- Seizures and head shaking.
- Chronic liver, pancreas, and urinary tract problems.

"These animals need improved diets, the right supplements, and to be helped with acupuncture and other natural means, but none of these good methods may work well unless you consider and rectify their hormonal mechanisms," Plechner says. "It's wonderful if you can enhance a system naturally that is suppressed, depressed, or screwed up some. I believe you can often do this with remarkable results. But many animals are too genetically defective, too far gone, and there is nothing you can do but replace the missing hormonal links—synthetically, with drugs. There is nothing there but a vacuum, and you can't enhance it, you can only fill it."

For many conditions, veterinary medicine relies intensely on a family of important synthetic cortisol drugs commonly called "steroids" or "cortisone" (such as Prednisone, Medrol, and Vetalog). They are anti-inflammatory and anti-itching agents that work well for a certain period of time, but when given in powerful pharmaceutical doses they can cause suppression of the adrenal glands and many side effects. If used properly, these drugs can keep many genetically flawed animals on an even keel, and indeed for some of them may be all that can keep them alive, says Plechner, adding that the key is using them properly, in doses that are physiologically relevant.

DETERMINING ACCURATE HORMONAL REPLACEMENT LEVELS

To determine accurate dosages, Plechner champions a blood test that, among other things, measures the level of cortisol an animal is producing. The test is called "the E-I One" test and is available to veterinarians at the National Veterinary Diagnostic Services, 23361 El Toro Rd., Suite 218, Lake Forest, CA 92630-6929 (phone: 949-859-3648). The criteria and range of normal values for the test were developed by Plechner.

The test monitors a critical range of hormonal and antibody activity: resting cortisol, total estrogen, testosterone, progesterone, T-3, T-4, IgA, IgM, and IgG. Comprehensive tests such as these are not done routinely by veterinarians.

Veterinarians tend not to measure cortisol and simply prescribe steroids that are often too strong or not appropriate. This results all too frequently in side effects. Plechner strongly recommends measuring the level of a patient's ability to produce natural cortisol and if a deficiency exists, to treat it *physiologically*.

"That means treating it at levels that are appropriate, and that usually means tiny amounts," he says. "You correct the body's own deficiency. You don't get the side effects then. I may correct a fifteen-pound cat totally out of sync with 1 milligram of Medrol, much less than a standard pharmaceutical dose of 4 milligrams."

One of the other important elements of the test is the measurement for total estrogen. Standard tests, by comparison, look only at a component of estrogen, called "estradiol." "I have found total estrogen to be a more accurate measurement of this one particular hormone," Plechner explains. "Estrogen can exert a dramatic blocking effect on cortisol and thyroid hormones, and just a slight variation out of the normal range is enough to cause a cascade of hormonal and immune complications."

Your veterinarian can also arrange for the laboratory to do a more comprehensive test (called "the E-I Two") that includes the E-I panel plus complete blood count and blood chemistry. "With this more elaborate test you can connect—and then correct—abnormalities in endocrine-immune activity to irregularities in organs or other systems in the body," according to Plechner. "Hormonal imbalances can be addressed by simple hormonal replacement therapy, which helps restore normal immune function. This is an important first step in therapy. It allows the veterinarian to make an accurate correction and manage it long-term. True genetic imbalances require lifelong management, in my opinion. Acquired imbalances can occur as a result of exposure to toxic chemicals, anesthesia, heavy metals, or pollutants. They may require only temporary management or, in some cases, management for a lifetime. This test is extremely beneficial in providing clues for intractable cases or where there have been substantial health problems early in an animal's life. It also has great benefit as a prevention tool in helping to determine which animals should or should not be bred."

Yet another test, called "the E-I Three," looks at four hormonal levels. Plechner recommends it for any individual considering the purchase of a kitten. The greater the hormonal imbalances revealed by this test, the greater the loss of control over the immune system and the earlier in an animal's life one sees health problems.

"If you find such imbalances, your choice is to put the cat on hormonal replacement or not accept the animal," Plechner says. "I would very much like to see breeders use passing marks in this test as criteria for future breeding of animals. Fortunately, I have increasing numbers of breeders who are using it. As they breed hormonally healthier animals they are finding fewer health problems in the offspring. This type of test offers a solution to the current nightmare. There is a great urgency to do something, and this is something we can all do."

Plechner says these special tests have allowed him, and other veterinarians who use them, to help animals who otherwise remain untreatable or who are walking time bombs just waiting to explode.

For individuals who may be philosophically opposed to using pharmaceutical drugs and synthetic hormones, Plechner says this: "Sometimes you can find natural options. Sometimes you can't. Recently, for instance, I have been successfully using a natural cortisone compound derived from soy. It is safe, effective and is readily absorbed in the body. Whether your veterinarian recommends a natural agent like this, or a synthetic one, the only way to save many of these pitiful creatures is to replace what is genetically missing in their bodies. I am all for correcting the diet, feeding the best possible food, and adding supplements, but do this, too. This is what the term 'holistic' should be all about. Looking at the whole picture. At least do these tests. Get the information."

The information, he says, provides something to think about for cases that may not respond to anything good, well-meaning, and natural you do for your cat.

TEST #2: THE BIO-NUTRITIONAL ANALYSIS

In his veterinary career, which has spanned three decades, Robert Goldstein, VMD, of Westport, Connecticut, has seen "the worst of the worst cases," many of them brought to him as a last resort after all other methods failed.

To help such seriously flawed animals, Goldstein, and his veterinarian brother, Martin, developed the Bio-Nutritional Analysis. The program utilizes data from an animal's blood tests, medical histories, and diagnoses to determine individual deficiencies and imbalances. With this information, an individualized strategy of effective diet and nutritional remedies is developed to address weaknesses and build up an ailing animal.

The Bio-Nutritional Analysis is offered to veterinarians through Antech Diagnostic Laboratories. Veterinarians can choose to have the nutritional analysis along with other standard blood tests performed by Antech. The program also offers an option of purchasing specific supplements that are recommended in the analysis for resale to pet owners. For more information, contact BioNutritional Diagnostics, Inc., at 800-670-0830.

"We have been using this analysis for more than twenty years, with impressive results, even for many cases where animals have been 'written off,'" says Goldstein. "Many have been animals so defective that even improved diet and natural remedies previously had little more than Band-Aid effects."

Obviously, he adds, "we must begin properly breeding animals with stronger immune systems and cut out this mass breeding just for the money. The kitty mills produce animals that are sicker and sicker at a younger age and more difficult for veterinarians to treat. This test provides a higher level of analysis than what is presently available, allowing practitioners to create an effective nutritional program for hard-to-manage patients."

✹ 16 ✹

Litter Box Tips

THANKS TO DRS. Nancy Scanlan, Lynne Friday, and Jean Hofve, for the following litter box advice:

- Find a litter box your cat likes. Clumping litter is very soft and cushy on their feet, so cats tend to like it. Declawed cats with tender feet will particularly like it. Some people feel that clumping litter is dangerous, that cats will eat it off their feet and get an intestinal blockage. This is possible but unlikely. The cat would have to consume a very large amount of litter for this to occur.

- Cleanliness is a feline obsession. The first commandment of litter box use is to clean the box regularly. Remember that a cat's sense of smell is ten times greater than ours and that supersmeller is only a few inches above the sand. Smell the box yourself. If it makes you sneeze, imagine what it's going to do to your kitties.

- Some cats won't enter a litter box with a lid. Lids keep the odor in. If you insist on a lidded box, you must be scrupulous about cleanliness. Stick *your* head in there. Does it smell clean? If it doesn't, that's probably why your cat may not want to go in.

- Some cats will not pee in their box because the litter smells too "perfumy." If you change your litter and then the animal doesn't want to use the box, go back to the original product with which the cat was well potty trained, and stick with it.

Baking soda spread over the bottom of the box can help get rid of some of the odor.

- If you have a litter box problem, try something different. If you have a lid, take the lid off. If you have clumping litter, try clay litter. If you can get the cat to use a cedar shaving box, all the better; it's ecological and compostable. But cats tend not to like the strong smell of cedar or other wood litters such as pine. Another option is a wheat-based clumping litter, such as Sweet Scoop, which is also biodegradable.

- Some older cats with crickety knees or sloppy style may miss the mark and pee or poop just outside the litter box. All four paws may be inside the box, but their rears will stick out over the edge and they'll make on the floor. If that's a problem, go to a hardware or general merchandise store and purchase a ten-inch Roughneck Tote container made by Rubbermaid. Fill it as you would any normal litter box. The container is about the same footprint as a litter box, only the sides are a bit taller. This allows the cat to get in readily but prevents the rear end from hanging over the side. Many plastic products give off an odor that cats don't like, but this product doesn't have an odor. It does have ridges on the bottom that make cleaning a bit of a challenge, but it is easier than constantly cleaning up "accidents."

- Ammonia compounds accompany the buildup of urine, which can contribute to runny eyes and noses and make cats more susceptible to respiratory conditions. As a preventive measure, pour out a thin layer of baking soda on the bottom of the inside of the box the next time you change the litter. Then add the litter material on top as usual. Don't mix the two.

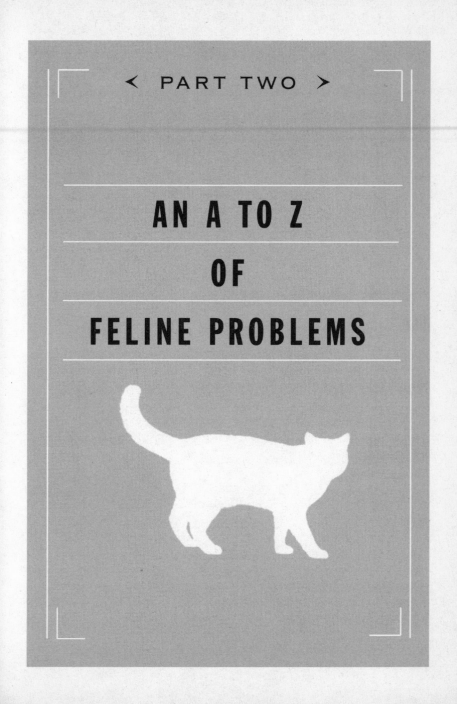

< PART TWO >

AN A TO Z

OF

FELINE PROBLEMS

INTRODUCTION
TO PART TWO

PART 2 IS divided alphabetically into the many different conditions that commonly affect cats. Under each condition you will find commentaries and recommendations from the veterinarians, with detailed instructions on how to use specific natural remedies. For general information on using natural products, refer to the appropriate chapter in part 1.

Many of the recommended supplements and remedies can be purchased at health food stores, pet stores, and drugstores or through natural pet product distributors or manufacturers. Some remedies, as noted in the text, are sold only to health professionals. You will have to ask your veterinarian to purchase such products for you.

For your convenience, the names and telephone numbers of manufacturers and distributors are included in the text to help you locate products not available in nearby stores. The addresses of these companies are also listed in appendix B.

If your cat is sick and does not improve after you try various recommendations and remedies presented in this book, be sure to see your veterinarian.

HOW TO GIVE YOUR CAT NATURAL REMEDIES

Cats are often difficult when it comes to taking medicines, supplements, or remedies. Unlike dogs, who will frequently gobble down a tablet or a capsule, cats tend not to be so cooperative. If there is ever a time to be sly in life, this is it! As one veterinarian commented, "The trouble with treating cats is treating cats."

In general, you should plan ahead so that giving a medicine or a supplement is not a battle royal, nor does it send your cat flying under the bed at the sight of you coming with an eyedropper or pill in your hand. This should be a bonding experience, not an ordeal.

It's important to know what you are going to do beforehand and do it quickly.

Follow up the administration of a remedy by patting and praising your cat for being cooperative. If you have persistent problems, and an extremely reluctant cat, ask your veterinarian to demonstrate an effective technique. Read the information here carefully. It can make a big difference in how successful you are.

Give nutritional supplements with food, unless directed otherwise. Herbal supplements should ideally be given apart from food. If your cat won't take the herbal product alone, mix it into the food.

If one form of the supplement or remedy is not easy to administer, try another. Remedies and supplements are available as powders, tablets, capsules, or liquids. Use the following guidelines for administering them:

- **Powdered supplements.** Mix into the food.

- **Capsules and tablets.** Give directly if not too large. Smear the pill in butter. That disguises the flavor and makes the pill slippery. Other options: Empty the contents of capsules into the food; crunch up tablets and mix into the food.

- **Pilling a cat.** Ask your veterinarian for a pill-popping dispenser, or pick one up from the pet store. To do it without a device, place the thumb and index finger of one hand under the cat's cheekbones and rotate the head upward so that the chin is pointing to the ceiling. This will relax the jaw. Gently open the jaw with your other hand. Then drop in the pill, straight down the middle and not into the cheek pockets on the sides. Do a fast poke, if needed, with your finger to push the pill down. Or use a pill gun. Let go of the cat's head so it can swallow. You will know the cat has swallowed the pill if it licks its nose. You don't have to hold the mouth shut. To help a pill go down faster, smear it in butter.

- **Liquids.** Give directly in the mouth or add to the food, as directed. To give orally, make a pouch on the side of the mouth by pulling out the lower lip slightly. Add the drops in the area of the molar teeth. Pets generally prefer the side route rather than a straight-down-the-middle, under-the-nose approach.

HOW TO GIVE NATURAL REMEDIES TO *VERY* FUSSY CATS

Cats fed two or more times a day tend to be more fussy than cats fed once. Following are some stealth tactics recommended by veterinarians:

- Try camouflaging the supplement in an aromatic or favored food. Examples: tuna oil, sardines, liver or liver juice, jars of baby meats, peanut butter, cottage cheese, or cream. Wrap or hide in a piece of solid food, such as a slice of turkey or chopped meat.

- If you use baby food, be sure the food contains no onion powder. Onions are toxic to cats and can cause anemia.

- Warm foods are more aromatic and palatable than cold or dry foods. Heating releases aromatic oils and spice flavors and offers more camouflage potential.

- Ask your veterinarian for a syringe that can be used to squirt supplements into the cat's mouth. Use a bit of liver juice or broth as the liquid base. Mix the supplement powder, capsule contents, or pulverized tablet into the juice or broth. Noni (morinda) is a tropical fruit from Hawaii with a great healing tradition. Cats generally don't mind the taste. Noni juice is another healthy base you can use for squirting supplements into cats.

GIVING THE PROPER DOSAGE TO YOUR CAT

The recommendations found throughout part 2 include dosage instructions. The dosages are generally to be given daily, unless otherwise noted.

For cats in particular it is a wise—and perhaps necessary—strategy to start low and go slow with natural remedies. If the taste of a supplement or herb is bitter or otherwise unpalatable, start with a very small dose, even a pinch or two. Stay at this level for several days or even a week. Then build up slowly to the recommended amount. Cats can be extremely fussy—and often reluctant—when it comes to new tastes and smells.

In the book you will sometimes encounter veterinarians recommending different dosages of the same supplement for a particular condition. If you have any doubts about how much to use, it is best to go with a lower dose and then, if needed, increase to a higher recommended level.

Dosages of individual flower essences and homeopathic remedies are generally the same—that is, the amount of the remedy you give is standard; only the frequency changes. General guidelines for these types of remedies are found in part 1. Follow the guidelines unless other instructions accompany a particular recommendation.

Vitamin C and the Bowel Tolerance Concept

Many holistic veterinarians recommend giving vitamin C to "bowel tolerance" therapeutic levels for certain conditions. What this means is slowly raising the amount of the supplement you give the animal in its food until you see the stool become soft. When you reach that level, reduce the amount slightly. Tolerance varies among individual animals. Try to give the vitamin C in divided doses throughout the day with food. The most economical and convenient form of vitamin C for these megadose quantities is buffered (nonacidic) sodium ascorbate crystals, which can be sprinkled onto food. Many years of clinical experience among both veterinarians and physicians who use megadoses of vitamin C demonstrate that the vitamin has powerful therapeutic properties when used in this manner. A quarter of a teaspoon of crystals is equal to 1,000 milligrams (1 gram).

ADVERSE REACTIONS TO NATURAL REMEDIES

Diarrhea or vomiting. If, after starting a particular remedy or supplement, an adverse reaction occurs, such as diarrhea or throwing up, stop the supplement. Sometimes you may avoid the reaction with a smaller dose. If that doesn't help, try a different supplement.

Some animals are particularly sensitive. In such cases it is prudent to introduce supplements at levels lower than the recommended dosages and increase the amount slowly.

Foaming at the mouth. This reaction may occur after administering a substance that is distasteful to the cat. A medication, supplement, or remedy may evoke foaming, an apparent attempt to expel the substance rather than swallow it. Cats have widely different foaming thresholds. There is no need to be concerned about the foaming itself, but if it happens, the cat may not be getting the full dosage. Moreover, it also forewarns likely long-term resistance ahead on the part of the cat. If you see foaming, use some of the methods detailed here to camouflage remedies in food the cat likes. Foaming that goes on for days may indicate an ulcer on the tongue or gums.

Some cats may foam because of the alcohol content in liquid homeopathic remedies, flower essences, and herbal tinctures. If this occurs, dilute the remedy in water or milk or simmer gently to release the alcohol. You can also try a different version of the remedy. For instance, homeopathics are also available in a lactose base, and tinctures in a glycerin base.

⚜ Abscesses ⚜

Abscesses are common and fairly obvious infections that develop after a cat is wounded by the claws or teeth of another cat. There is a swelling where the injury has occurred. The cat may be feverish or sit off in a corner and not eat.

The swelling that develops under the site of the puncturelike wound is hard at first and then softens as the abscess forms. The area of the swelling may be painful and hot.

Generally you may not notice the abscess until it opens and starts to drain. If the cat is eating and otherwise feels good, the crisis is over. Just keep the wound clean and let the animal's immune system handle it. A healthy cat should have plenty of antibodies to deal with the germs. Left alone like this, the animal may not be prone to abscesses from bite wounds in the future. In most cases the abscess will heal by itself.

However, if the cat is sick for a day, not eating, or lethargic, take it to a veterinarian. That means the cat isn't dealing well with the abscess.

There are many reasons for supplementing your animal with a good multi-vitamin mineral formula. One is that it helps fortify the immune system. You may not be able to keep your cat from getting into fights, but you can keep its immune system strong so that it is less likely to develop an infection if injured.

If it does become wounded during battle, several homeopathic remedies are highly effective for mustering the animal's own healing resources against abscesses without the need for medication.

HOMEOPATHIC REMEDIES
(See chapter 9 for general dosage guidelines.)

High-Strength Hepar Sulph—Karen Bentley, DVM
The remedy Hepar sulphuris at a high potency of 200C works well in the case of a fresh abscess and eight out of ten times can prevent the problem from developing into a putrid mess. Use this remedy when the cat comes in with a swelling that hasn't burst yet. The remedy is available in health food stores or homeopathic pharmacies.

DOSAGE
• 1 dose only.

Low-Strength Hepar Sulph—Charles Loops, DVM
If the abscess is large, feels hot, and is sensitive to the touch, and you want it to open up and drain, use Hepar sulphuris at the low potency of 6 or 12X. If the abscess feels hot and is sensitive to the touch, but is not very swollen, use the higher-potency Hepar sulphuris 30C.

If the abscess is without heat and is not sensitive to the touch, use Silicea 30C.

These remedies should take care of the abscess. If you don't see improvement in twenty-four to forty-eight hours with one remedy, try the other.

DOSAGE
• **Hepar sulphuris 6 or 12X:** Several times daily.

- **Hepar sulphuris 30C:** Once or twice for a day.
- **Silicea 30C:** Once or twice for a day.

Lachesis—Ron Carsten, DVM

I have treated many cat abscesses successfully with Lachesis, the homeopathic remedy made from the poison of the bushmaster snake. The sooner after the injury you give the remedy, the quicker the results. Lachesis often works by itself and eliminates the need for antibiotics. Monitor the situation carefully. If the animal doesn't respond, isn't eating or drinking, and becomes progressively depressed, see a veterinarian immediately. Other things could be going on.

DOSAGE
- If you can obtain the high-potency 1M remedy, give it one time. Otherwise use Lachesis 30C three times daily for three days.

Ledum Plus Hot Packs—Jean Hofve, DVM

If you see a puncture wound and know your cat has just been in a fight, use the homeopathic remedy Ledum 30C. That will head off most wounds developing into abscesses.

"Hot packs" are useful. Take a washcloth, dip it in warm water, and apply it to the affected area. Once the cat gets over the original shock that you are up to something, it will probably just sit back and enjoy the experience because it feels good. The "hot pack" draws circulation into the wound area and helps prevent abscesses from developing.

DOSAGE
- **Ledum 30C:** Two or three times during the first twenty-four hours.

⚓ Arthritis ⚓

Among our companion animals, dogs are more prone to arthritis, but yes, cats get it, too. Arthritis may develop as a degenerative condition from years of wear and tear, causing pain, stiffness, lessened activity, and trouble going up and down stairs.

Cats are very jumpy critters and very flexible. Damage to the joints, which act as shock absorbers between bones, can occur as a result of small injuries that you may not notice at the time. These minor traumas pile up over the years and undermine the integrity of the cartilage and soft connective tissue of the joints. Eventually the damage causes sufficient discomfort to slow down the cat.

Most older animals have some kind of arthritic back problem whether you can see it on X-ray or not.

Conventional medications for arthritis are used very cautiously by veterinarians. This is because cats cannot tolerate many of these medicines, including nonsteroidal anti-inflammatory drugs, aspirin, and acetaminophen.

Along with natural remedies, holistic veterinarians typically recommend acupuncture and/or chiropractic treatment for animals with arthritis.

HERBS

Chinese Herbal Formula—Joseph Demers, DVM

Du Huo Jisheng Wan, a classical Chinese herbal formula, works very well for my feline arthritis cases. The product comes in tiny black pills and is available at Chinese groceries or pharmacies. The formula contains ginger, cinnamon, angelica, Chinese foxglove, and licorice root and acts to tonify the liver, kidney, and blood. The Chinese say it dispels wind and dampness in the joints, lower back, and knees that cause weakness, pain, and stiffness.

The formula is as effective as other drugs I used previously for animals who are stiff and having a hard time getting up or down. Often you see improvement within a few days. Use for one to three weeks and then as needed.

DOSAGE
- 2 or 3 pills twice a day. Smear the pills with butter for taste and to help them slide down the throat.

Ayurvedic Herbal Combination—Tejinder Sodhi, DVM

Boswellia (Indian frankincense) and ashwaganda (winter cherry), two very well-known herbs from the Ayurvedic healing tradition of India, provide excellent relief. Significant improvement occurs within fourteen to twenty-one days in a majority of cases, although very severe conditions may take up to three months.

I recommend the liquid form of these herbs for cats, available through Ayush Herbs (800-925-1371). Both are glycerine-based products.

Boswellia is a potent anti-inflammatory, with much research demonstrating significant relief of pain and stiffness in arthritic patients. It effectively shrinks inflamed tissue, the underlying cause of pain in many conditions. It also increases blood supply to affected areas and promotes repair of local blood vessels damaged by proliferating inflammation.

Ashwaganda is also a powerful anti-inflammatory and contains a natural compound that exerts an anabolic effect in the body. This means that it can help strengthen atrophied muscles around diseased joints. Ashwaganda acts on the musculoskeletal and nervous systems, generating energy and vitality. It has an adaptogenic action somewhat like ginseng, meaning that it helps counteract the effects of stress.

DOSAGE
- **Boswellia and ashwaganda:** 10 drops per ten pounds of body weight twice daily for each herbal.

NUTRITIONAL SUPPLEMENTS

Potent Antioxidant Supplement—Thomas Van Cise, DVM

Dismutase, a whole-food antioxidant supplement prepared from specially grown wheat and soy sprouts, is a potent natural agent for arthritis. The product, made by BioVet International (800-788-1084), usually generates improvement within three weeks, but it can sometimes happen faster, in a matter of days. You frequently see older animals with renewed energy. There are no side effects.

Dismutase scavenges free radicals, molecular renegades in the body that contribute to accelerated aging and disease. The action of the product helps reduce inflammation and the destruction of cartilage.

The supplement will not remake the joint. But there won't be any discomfort, and the flexibility and energy it generates is often phenomenal. Dismutase tastes like dry bread. I have used the flavored veterinary version of Dismutase but find that the human version works better.

DOSAGE
- For the vast majority of cats, 1 tablet works well. If you have a large cat, you can try 2 tablets and see if there is added improvement. Preferably give on an empty stomach. Some cats will eat the tablet, others won't. If the cat won't take it, and you don't want to pill the cat, than grind it into a powder and mix into the food.

Success with Cosequin and NuCat—Jean Hofve, DVM

Cosequin, a neutraceutical formulation made by Nutramax Laboratories (800-925-5187; sold through veterinarians), works fabulously. The product contains glucosamine hydrochloride and chondroitin sulfate, two substances that resemble natural compounds found in healthy cartilage tissue.

NuCat, from VetriScience (800-882-9993; sold through veterinarians), contains green-lipped mussels, which is another very helpful compound. One older cat I put on this product started jumping up on her owner's dryer again, something she hadn't done in years.

With either one of these formulations you should see results within three to four weeks. These are palliative treatments, but they work well to make the joint fluid more slippery, and that reduces the amount of inflammation in the area of the joint. With either product, follow label instructions.

Vitamins, DLPA, SOD, Glucosamine—Nancy Scanlan, DVM

For mild cases, use vitamins E and C and dl-phenylalanine (DLPA), an amino acid that diminishes pain and is especially useful where animals have hind leg weakness. These three supplements also work well for more muscle-related conditions or where there is no clear X-ray evidence of arthritis.

For more severe cases or when the animal isn't responding to E, C, and DLPA, add sodium oxide dismutase (SOD), an antioxidant with good anti-inflammatory properties; or any one or more of the popular antiarthritis supplements such as glucosamine sulfate, chondroitin sulfate, and green-lipped mussels.

Each of these supplements acts in a somewhat different way, and often you don't know for sure which one is going to be the pivotal element providing the most significant relief. Remember that each animal is individual. Some will do better on glucosamine sulfate than on chondroitin; others will benefit more from the green-lipped mussels.

Whichever supplements you administer, don't give them all at once at full strength. Start slowly so that you don't overload the system and cause diarrhea. If diarrhea occurs, reduce the supplements, particularly vitamin C and SOD.

I usually see improvement in about two weeks, but it can happen earlier or later, up to a month. I cannot predict the speed of improvement from an X-ray or the animal's condition when first brought in. However, one way to accelerate healing and ease pain is acupuncture with a qualified veterinary specialist. Acupuncture is wonderful for these conditions. You can also help with regular massaging (refer to chapter 13).

DOSAGE

- When an animal improves on this program, reduce dosage of the supplements, such as going from twice to once a day. Some animals, however, may require a full dose on a long-term basis. If an animal starts to show renewed signs of arthritis when you reduce the supplement, return to the higher levels.

- Use the lower recommended levels for smaller cats.

- **Vitamin C:** 125 to 250 milligrams twice daily.

- **Vitamin E:** 50 to 100 IU once a day.

- **SOD:** 100 milligrams once a day. If you don't see improvement, increase to twice daily. Go slow so as not to cause diarrhea.

- **DLPA:** 100 milligrams twice daily.

- **Glucosamine sulfate:** 100 to 250 milligrams twice daily.

- **Chondroitin sulfate:** 100 to 200 milligrams twice daily.

- **Green-lipped mussels:** 150 milligrams once a day.

Relief from Sea Cucumber—Carolyn Blakey, DVM

For any animal with joint problems, I have had consistent and long-term good results with SeaCuMax, a sea cucumber supplement from Maine (made by Coastside Bio Resources, 207-367-2297). This is an all-natural product containing natural compounds (including chondroitin sulfate) that generate a powerful anti-inflammatory effect. I recommend it any time there is a sign of discomfort in the joints. That could mean stiffness, slowness to move, an animal not wanting to move as far as it used to, or limping.

When I usually see a case, there is already some erosion of the joint health. Most of these animals don't turn around to healthy joints again. But we can help them substantially with a product like this. Over the years I have used many natural products, as well as synthetic supplements such as glucosamine sulfate. I feel this particular brand of sea cucumber has given me the best results to date during the three years I have used it.

DOSAGE
- Follow label instructions. Available in powder or capsule form and also as a "jerky" treat.

⚓ Asthma ⚓

This condition is frequently seen in cats, and more so now than previously, veterinarians say.

Asthma is an inflammation of the airways leading into the lungs.

The inflammation creates spasm, a buildup of clogging mucus, and a contraction of surrounding muscles. The result in cats, just as in people, is difficult breathing.

Airborne pollen allergens are often involved in asthma, as is constant exposure to dust and mold. Remember that cats live close to the ground, where dust and mold collect. Food allergies and chemical sensitivities, usually overlooked, can also be major culprits.

"The increase in asthmatic cats is pollution related," says Nancy Scanlan, DVM. "I see many cats suffering from the gases emitted by synthetic carpets, particularly when the carpets are new. Some owners have told me that the asthma problem has cleared up when carpets were removed. People are frequently affected by carpets as well."

Cortisone and antihistamine medications are usually prescribed for asthmatic cats.

HERBS

Minor Blue Dragon Plus Acupuncture—Nancy Scanlan, DVM
The combination of acupuncture along with Chinese herbs offers a powerful therapeutic 1-2 punch. Using these two methods, I can invariably make animals more comfortable and cut down their requirement for medication. In mild cases I am able to eliminate their drugs altogether.

The Chinese herbal formula I use is a human product called Minor Blue Dragon, available through health professionals and veterinarians. I obtain my supply from Health Concerns (800-233-9355).

I recommend using this formula under the guidance of a veterinarian with herbal knowledge because it contains the herb ma huang. Ma huang is the source of ephedra, a powerful bronchodilating agent that has been synthesized for chemical drugs used by asthmatics. If an animal is already taking ephedra drugs on a regular basis, you have to be careful when adding what may be an additional source of ephedra. That's why it is best done with a veterinarian.

With this effective formula, I am able to reduce the amount of cortisone, or eliminate it totally, in every case. If asthmatic attacks persist, they are always less severe and animals don't require hospitalization nearly as often as they used to.

DOSAGE
- Give twice daily. Small cats, 1/4 tablet; larger cats, 1/2 tablet.

More Minor Blue Dragon Success—Nino Aloro, DVM

I have had excellent results with Naturafed, a Chinese herbal formula from Pacific BioLogic (800-869-8783). This human product, containing pinellia, ma huang, cinnamon, peony root, schizandra, nettles, licorice root, and wild ginger, is based on a 1,200-year-old Chinese formula known as the Minor Blue Dragon for mild asthma.

About 80 percent of cats are responsive, and I use it except for the most severe cases. Usually within a week you see improvement. Animals are more comfortable, able to breathe easier and with less coughing. This product helps minimize the need for medication. I have cats taking it for more than five years, and they are doing well.

DOSAGE
- 1 capsule twice a day.

HOMEOPATHIC REMEDIES
(See chapter 9 for general dosage guidelines.)

Ipecacuanha for Acute Attacks—Charles Loops, DVM

Two homeopathic remedies help to relieve acute difficulty of breathing—Ipecacuanha or Carbo vegetabilis at a 6C potency. Try the Ipecacuanha first. If it doesn't work, try the other remedy. If neither one resolves the crisis, bring the animal to a veterinarian.

Frequently this problem develops a month or so after a vaccination shot. The vaccine may trigger stress in the cat's body. If there is a genetic weakness in the lungs, the stress can manifest as asthma.

DOSAGE
- Either remedy can be given every hour for a few doses.

MIXED AND MISCELLANEOUS APPROACHES

Oxygen for Easier Breathing—Thomas Van Cise, DVM

I recommend an oral stabilized oxygen product for any lung or allergic condition. Many are available in health food stores. The brand I use is Earth Bounty Oxy-Max from Matrix Health Products (800-736-5609). This product oxygenates the whole body, including the lungs, and helps to clear out toxins generated by allergies.

You will typically see improved breathing within days. If you have an older pet, or an animal who has been on a lot of medication, such as steroids for allergies, then it will take longer, maybe two weeks.

DOSAGE
- Give twice daily on food: 6 to 8 drops for an eight-pound cat; up to 10 drops for a cat fifteen pounds or more.

Herbs, Homeopathics, and Supplements—Roger DeHaan, DVM

Instead of the typical cortisone treatments, which can be detrimental to health over the long term, I suggest a combination of remedies that has worked very well. It is also helpful for seasonal pollen allergies and almost any allergic condition. Generally, within a week or two animals are much improved. You'll see less wheezing, sneezing, and difficulty in breathing.

Each of the following remedies in the program is available through Holistic Veterinary Services (218-846-9112):

- Licorice root, an herb that supports the adrenal glands. These organs produce cortisol, the body's natural stress hormone (Prednisone and other steroid drugs are pharmaceutical versions of cortisol). The adrenals become burdened and overworked when the system is exposed to constant allergenic substances. I use a liquid form of licorice root made by Nature's Sunshine.

- Allerplex, made by Standard Process, is a whole-food supplement with raw adrenal and lung glandulars. This product supports affected tissue and also acts as a natural antibiotic.

- Asthma Homeopathic or Dust & Mold Homeopathic, combination homeopathic remedies made by Nature's Sunshine. You can use these or any allergy-related homeopathic remedies available in health food stores.

DOSAGE
- **Licorice root:** 5 drops twice a day in the food for three weeks. Then for five days a week as long as needed.

- **Allerplex:** 1/4 tablet twice a day in food.

- **Asthma Homeopathic or Dust & Mold Homeopathic:** 3 to 4 drops several times a day.

⍋ Bad Breath ⍋

Halitosis (bad breath) is generally caused by two things: dental problems or poor digestion.

NUTRITIONAL SUPPLEMENTS

Digestive Aids—Lynne Friday, DVM
First, look in the mouth. The problem may be bad teeth or gums, cancer of the mouth, or bones stuck between teeth.

If the mouth isn't the problem, give your pet digestive aids such as digestive enzymes, ginger snaps, or Chlorets. I use Chlorowin, made by Wintec Inc. (314-257-5400), a digestive aid with chlorophyll, mint, and liver for palatability. The product helps combat bad breath as well as odors during heat. Another good supplement is chlorella, available in health food stores.

DOSAGE
- **Chlorowin:** Follow label instructions.

MIXED AND MISCELLANEOUS APPROACHES

Enzymes Plus Green Vegetables—Carvel Tiekert, DVM

Cats by nature have bad breath. This could be in part because they eat more meat. But they do not have highly efficient digestive systems. One reason dogs like to eat cat stool is that cats are inefficient digesters of protein, and dogs like predigested protein.

If the teeth are clean, purchase pet digestive enzymes for your animal. The enzymes help the animal break down and absorb food. Green vegetables in the diet are also helpful. The veggies contain, among other things, lots of chlorophyll, a natural detoxifier. Prepare them lightly steamed and smeared with butter (the butter is a good flavor enhancer).

If halitosis persists, see a veterinarian. There may be a liver problem.

Peppermint Oil—Jan Bellows, DVM

Peppermint oil, available in health food stores, has a minty scent and is antibacterial and anti-inflammatory. It will not cure periodontal disease (see the section on dental health), but it will help with the breath. Other options for bad breath include natural toothpastes, baking soda, lemon juice, and finely ground rubbed sage.

DOSAGE
- **Peppermint oil:** Add a few drops of this or spearmint essential oil to a cup of distilled water and use as a mouth spray.

FOOD AND SPECIAL DIETS

Food Allergies?—Alfred Plechner, DVM

Bad breath, without dental disease, may mean you are looking at a problem of food that doesn't agree with an animal. The immune cells in the mouth are overreacting to foodstuffs and you get a kind of "dermatitis of the mouth" and a bad smell. A red flare, or line, above the teeth, or even an entire oral cavity that appears inflamed, is a major sign that the problem is being caused by glandular or immune system imbalances that often generate food allergies and other disorders (see section on food allergies; also see chapter 15 on what to do when nothing seems to work).

⚜ Behavioral Problems ⚜

See also: Stress, Food Allergies

Stress, boredom, and changes in a cat's environment can lead to emotional disturbances. Consider these possibilities when confronted with new, strange behavior.

Many holistic veterinarians recommend flower essences, unique natural remedies that are actually derived from flowers, to alleviate behavioral problems. Homeopathics are also frequently used.

Look to your cat's diet as a possible source of nervousness, hyperactivity, and other unusual behavior. Regularly feeding poor-quality food laced with chemical additives always has the potential to cause problems, physical or behavioral. Food additives can be major behavioral triggers. So, too, can certain foods that act as allergens. Refer to the food chapters in part 1 to see how you can feed your cat a better diet.

If the simple approaches described here don't work, consult with an animal behaviorist or your veterinarian. Deeper issues may be involved that require professional attention.

FLOWER ESSENCES
(See chapter 10 on flower essences for dosing instructions.)

Jealousy, Fear, and Grief—Jean Hofve, DVM

- **Jealousy.** Cats are sensitive critters and easily become jealous or upset when they sense interference in their territory. Take a situation, for instance, where a cat and its human female companion have been sole occupants in an apartment. Now, suddenly, a boyfriend appears on the scene. One night the boyfriend throws his leather jacket on the chair. The next morning it is full of cat urine. That's the work of an upset cat.

  I developed a combination of flower essences called Peacemaker that reduces aggression, discord, and jealousy between cats and facilitates the acceptance of a new relationship or family member on the scene, whether it involves a human adult, child, baby, or another animal. Often when a new cat is introduced into the household, the old cat will start spraying, howling, or fighting with the new arrival. This formula will help defuse that situation as well.

The liquid remedy includes Holly, for jealousy; Beech, to increase tolerance; Walnut, for change; and Willow, for resentment. Peacemaker is available through the Internet from Flower Essence Therapy for Animals at www.spirit essence.com.

- **Grief.** Solace is another flower combination remedy I developed (available through the Internet Web site above) for grieving animals. It includes Water Violet, the major essence for grief, and Honeysuckle, for animals (and humans) living in the past who indulge in wishing that things were as they used to be.

  The remedy helps not just cats, but also dogs, birds, and even horses who go to a new home after the death of an owner and are just not adjusting well, or for situations where a companion animal has died. One cat I treated had lived in a house for many years with a dog. After the dog died, the cat constantly went to the door, waiting for its companion to come in from the yard. The cat was distraught and pining. In cases such as these, flower remedies work quickly to reestablish emotional equilibrium and overcome obvious grief.

- **Fear.** Flower remedies work quickly for fearful animals, particularly the combination of Rescue Remedy, Mimulus, and Aspen. These remedies are available at health food stores.

  I recall the case of one cat who had been adopted from the local Humane Society. After being installed in its new house, it remained under a dresser and came out only in the quiet of the night to eat, drink, and use the litter box. This went on for two weeks. Within two hours of a single dose of the combined remedy, the cat was out exploring the premises. I have had many people call me the next day after starting this combination and say it's as if they have a new cat.

To make the combination remedy, do the following:

1. Purchase the individual bottles of Rescue Remedy, Mimulus, and Aspen.
2. Add 2 drops from each bottle into a clean 1-ounce bottle filled with spring water.
3. Use the remedy according to the general directions in the chapter on flower essences.

Walnut for Upset—Carolyn Blakey, DVM

For any major, upsetting changes in the environment of a cat, Walnut is very helpful. Use this remedy, for instance, when there is a new addition to the household or when a move or a death has occurred.

Sad Cats and Sad Pet Owners—Donna Starita Mehan, DVM

Zinnia puts back playfulness and lightheartedness in animals and even their sad human companions. I use the product made by the Flower Essence Society (800-736-9222). This is a wonderful remedy for all creatures who are depressed or heavy and who have forgotten how to have a good time. People say it brings back smiles to their faces, humor to their hearts, and friskiness to their animals.

DOSAGE
- 1 drop twice a day in water or food, or rub a drop on the ear of the cat.

HOMEOPATHIC REMEDIES
(See chapter 9 for general dosage guidelines.)

Ignatia for Grief—Michele Yasson, DVM

Any time a cat loses a companion animal or human, it can experience grief just as we do. Ignatia, a dependable homeopathic remedy for grief, is often helpful.

DOSAGE
- **Ignatia 30C:** For older cats, a single dose usually works. For middle-aged cats, twice a day for two days, if needed; and for younger cats, three times a day for two days.

Hyperactivity/Noise Sensitivity—Roger DeHaan, DVM

For animals who are hyper or who become agitated by loud noises, there are a number of good natural remedies that work in a large percentage of cases. They include the following:

- **CalmStress,** a homeopathic combination remedy from Dr. Goodpet (800-222-9932).

- **Aconite 30X,** a single homeopathic remedy.

Often these remedies will calm an animal immediately, after a single dose, or within a few days of giving them two or three times a day. At least try them for a month. If you don't see results by then, you need to consult with a veterinarian to sort out the causes. But these remedies are good places to start.

NUTRITIONAL SUPPLEMENTS

B Complex—Carvel Tiekert, DVM

Many animals can be helped with just a regular stress vitamin B-complex formula alone, particularly if the problem is antisocial behavior such as aggression and short temper.

Try the supplement for a month. It will either help—or not help—within that time. I have found that this simple, inexpensive supplement works in about 30 to 40 percent of cases.

But be sure to get rid of the food with chemicals, which can be a big trigger.

DOSAGE
- One-quarter of a 50-milligram capsule or tablet a day.

⚜ Cancer ⚜

Cancer involves an uncontrolled growth of cells on or inside the body. Among pets it is a common disease. The incidence of disease increases with age and, according to the American Veterinary Medical Association, accounts for almost half of the deaths of pets over the age of ten years. Dogs are more often affected than are cats; however, tumors are more often malignant in cats.

The most common types of feline cancers are the following:

- Lymphomas, malignant enlargements of one or numerous lymph nodes.
- Breast tumors. Eighty-five percent are malignant.
- Abdominal tumors.
- Skin tumors.

Interestingly, many veterinarians interviewed for this book expressed concern about seeing more younger animals than ever before developing cancer.

"When I started in practice more than twenty-five years ago, cancer was a disease of older animals," says Robert Goldstein, VMD, who regards cancer as an epidemic disease among pets. "Now you see it regularly when they are one, two, and three."

The increase in cancer is attributed by holistic veterinarians to genetic weaknesses fostered by contemporary breeding practices along with poor diet, medications, chemical dips and additives, vaccines, and stress.

Holistic medicine regards cancer as a failure of the immune system. It is seen as a systemic disease that may appear locally as skin tumors in one patient or breast cancer in another. But the underlying problem, in the holistic viewpoint, is a failure of the body's defenses to stop abnormal mutating cells from growing rapidly.

Just as their human medicine counterparts, veterinary oncologists (animal doctors specializing in cancer treatments) recommend chemotherapy, radiation, and surgery. For some forms of cancer, surgery is the best option. Skin tumors, for instance, can often be eliminated cleanly by surgery, especially when treated early. Drugs and radiation are also beneficial when used appropriately. For lymphomas, chemotherapy can be very effective and should be considered as an option.

Natural healing methods, unlike conventional treatments, are not invasive. They emphasize strengthening a weakened immune system and can be used in two ways:

1. In combination with standard treatments to reduce side effects and speed healing. Animals undergoing chemotherapy or surgery tend to do much better.

2. As the major modality, under the care of a holistic veterinarian, and bypassing standard therapies.

Cats tend to be more difficult to treat than dogs, says Nancy Scanlan, DVM, author of a book on cancer treatments for pets. "The problem is that they are less willing to take herbs and supplements and also that cat livers do not detoxify chemotherapy agents as well as dog livers do."

Alternative treatments are highly varied and multifaceted. As Roger DeHaan, DVM, points out, "There is as yet no 'magic bullet' that kills cancer cells. The holistic approach tries to build up the immune system and improve nutrition. Any time you do these things you are going to help the animal—or the person—combat cancer. The normal pet's body is equipped to kill or discard unhealthy cells. My goal is to fortify this natural ability. I believe this is the best way to tackle cancer."

The following commentaries and programs provide useful general information on how to build up your animal to help in its fight against cancer. These insights may also provide new hope and additional recourse for situations in which a veterinarian says there is nothing more that can be done. Keep in mind, however, that cancer is a life-threatening condition. Don't try to treat it on your own. If you decide to pursue a natural healing approach, look for a qualified holistic veterinarian near you who can individualize a program for your particular cat and the type of cancer it has. This offers the very best chance of extending and improving the quality of life or enhancing the possibility of recovery.

General points made by the veterinarians include these:

- **Think prevention.** Does your pet have a carcinogenic lifestyle? Does it eat a diet filled with poor-quality ingredients and chemical additives, and is it exposed to toxic flea preparations and multiple medications? We need to correct the diet, reduce chemical exposure in an animal's environment, and try to resolve stress problems *before* cancer manifests and the major organs of the body are compromised. Cancer generally has more than one cause.

- **Good nutrition is critical.** Food as medicine is particularly important for very sick animals. An anticancer diet excludes commercial pet food, veterinarians say. It requires a homemade diet emphasizing fresh, wholesome food, and lightly steamed vegetables (see chapter 6). Avoid chemical additives. "Unless this is done," says Joseph Demers, DVM, "I don't think affected animals have a fighting chance."

- **Use of supplements.** Holistic veterinarians usually recommend multiple vitamin/mineral nutritional supplements to strengthen the immune system, plus extra vitamin C and other antioxidants. The recommendations offered here can be used in virtually all cases, even if your animal is being treated conventionally. Select one particular veterinarian's program and work with it. Note that different veterinarians recommend some of the same supplements at somewhat different dosages. Start supplementing at a lower dose and work up slowly to recommended levels.

- **Stress weakens the body.** It depletes important cancer-fighting vitamins, such as vitamin C, and interferes with digestion and the nervous system. Stress reduces the power of the immune system to kill or neutralize cancer. (See discussion on stress later in the book.)

- **Last resort.** Holistic veterinarians say they tend to see animals who have been previously treated with chemotherapy and who are then brought to them as a last resort. "Even though they may be near the end we can frequently improve their quality of life for the time that is left," says Tejinder Sodhi, DVM.

HERBS

Essiac—Nino Aloro, DVM

One of the herbs I routinely use in my individualized approach to cancer is Essiac. I use the capsule form. I find that this herb helps promote recovery and when taken long-term acts as a preventive against recurrent tumors.

Essiac is an herbal combination developed by a Canadian nurse, Rene Caisse, who for a period of more than fifty years treated many hundreds of patients with cancer. Essiac is Caisse spelled backward. Caisse never made her formula public in her lifetime. She said the formula had been given to her by a patient who had been cured from breast cancer by an Indian herbalist. The four main ingredients in Essiac are burdock, Indian rhubarb, sorrel, and slippery elm. In the 1970s Essiac was tested at two U.S. cancer institutions and said to offer no anticancer activity. According to Ralph Moss, Ph.D., in *Cancer Therapy: The Independent Consumer's Guide to Non-Toxic Treatment & Prevention* (Equinox Press, Brooklyn, N.Y., 1992), "the mixture remains worth investigating, not just because of persistent anecdotal reports, but because most of its identifiable components have individually shown anticancer properties in independent tests."

More on Essiac—Michele Yasson, DVM

For any animal being treated for cancer either conventionally or holistically, Essiac tea is an excellent natural remedy to add to the program. It acts as a blood cleanser. It tends to increase elimination—you may see more voluminous stool. It also stimulates the appetite, which is desirable in cancer cases, and increases the immune system's effectiveness against cancer cells.

I recommend a tea called Whisker's Own Rednop Essiac, a blend of Essiac plus pau d'arco and red clover blossom, prepared by Whisker's Holistic Pet Products (800-944-7537). Follow label instructions. It comes in a powder form that you make into a tea and then administer by dropper down the animal's throat. Essiac tea is mildly bitter. When an animal is fighting a serious illness such as cancer, some people are reluctant to force a liquid medication on animals. Although I prefer the tea, there is an alternative—a freeze-dried crystal form of Essiac that can be put right into the food. It is called E Tea and is made by Nature's Sunshine (800-223-8225).

DOSAGE
- **Whisker's Essiac:** Follow label instructions.

- **E Tea:** One-quarter of the human dose on the label.

NUX VOMICA FOR CHEMOTHERAPY

For animals receiving chemotherapy treatments, I recommend the homeopathic remedy Nux vomica to help the body cope more effectively against the toxicity of the drugs. Chemotherapy often generates adverse side effects. As the treatment progresses, animals are more likely to become sick and develop vomiting or diarrhea. Nux vomica can make a big difference. It can be given at any time during the treatment program.

DOSAGE
- If the side effects are not severe, give a single dose of Nux vomica 30C immediately after the chemo treatment. If side effects are severe, give twice a day for two days.

HOMEOPATHIC REMEDIES

Homeopathy vs. Cancer—Charles Loops, DVM

Seventy percent of my cases involve cancer. Homeopathy offers an effective alternative to conventional approaches for this devastating disease. In general, you can accomplish with homeopathy the same results obtained with chemotherapy, radiation, and surgical treatments. Often we can accomplish more. However, I strongly recommend that you consult with an experienced veterinary homeopath because the remedies used must be skillfully individualized.

We do get cures with homeopathy. More than 50 percent of animals go into remission if treated early enough, yet even with more advanced cases we have results that are similar to invasive therapies, but without the side effects. In general, the tumors that respond the best to chemotherapy and radiation are the same that respond to homeopathy.

In my opinion, homeopathy helps pain better than any drug. The animal will feel much better right up to the end. Homeopathy seems to ensure a dying process that is more natural, as compared with the effects of a drug treatment protocol. Often with homeopathy we are able to extend the lives of animals given only a short time to live by other veterinarians. This is because homeopathy uplifts the animal's life force.

In addition to homeopathics, there are many other remedies you can apply to strengthen an animal diagnosed with cancer. I have found the following to be particularly helpful.

PRODUCTS AND DOSAGE

- **Chinese astragalus:** This herb is an excellent immune stimulant that can be used indefinitely on a daily basis. It is available as a herbal tincture or in capsule form. Give 3 drops or 1 capsule twice daily.

- **Grapeseed extract:** 1 milligram per pound of body weight twice daily.

- **Multi-vitamin mineral:** Pro VitaMix or other quality formulas available through Morrill's New Directions (800-368-5057). Follow label instructions.

- **Vitamin C:** 500 milligrams twice a day.

- **Vitamin E:** 200 IU daily.

- **Omega-3 fatty acid fish oils (such as salmon):** 1,000 milligrams daily.

MIXED AND MISCELLANEOUS APPROACHES

Antioxidants and Chinese Herbs—Nancy Scanlan, DVM

(Note: Scanlan has written a comprehensive book on cancer in pets—*Cancer, All the Options, A Wholistic View of Cancer Therapy*, available through Hibridge Press, San Jose, California, at 800-860-9422. This book offers the latest information on all cancer treatments—conventional and holistic—for dogs and cats.)

Whatever course of treatment you choose, support it with a strong supplement program to protect and reinforce the animal's immune system. Antioxidants, such as vitamins C and E, and coenzyme Q$_{10}$, will accomplish this, in addition to exerting specific anti-cancer benefits. These supplements should be a major part of any cancer program. Antioxidants also offer protection against the side effects of chemotherapy.

Omega-3 fatty acids, as found in fish liver oils (containing eicosapentaenoic or decosahexaenoic acids), also give nutritional support. Animal studies have shown they inhibit tumor growth and metastasis.

IP-6 is a form of inositol, a B-complex vitamin, that has promise as another antioxidant.

I also recommend two Chinese herbal formulas made for humans that have anticancer properties. They are extremely helpful in dealing with cancer in animals. Both are made by Health Concerns (800-233-9355) and are available through health professionals or veterinarians. I use Power Mushrooms, one of the formulas, for any kind of cancer as well as to boost immunity in animals with weak defenses. I have used Regeneration, the other formula, for its anticancer properties as well as its ability to help counteract the side effects of chemotherapy. These products come in tablet form and do not have a taste that a cat will like. If you can't pill your cat (see how to give remedies at the beginning of part 2), Chinese herbal formulas can be difficult to give. They don't taste good!

DOSAGE

- **Vitamin C:** Go to bowel tolerance. Sicker animals tolerate more than healthier animals. Their bodies need more. (See note to reader at beginning of part 2 on how to give vitamin C in this manner.)

- **Vitamin E:** 50 IU once a day. You can safely double the dose in serious cases.

- **Coenzyme Q$_{10}$:** 20 milligrams. You can use higher amounts, but watch for possible signs of gastric upset or decreased appetite.

- **Omega-3 fatty acids:** 250 milligrams daily. Do not use omega-3 fatty acids that are combined with omega-6 oils.

- **IP-6:** 50 to 100 milligrams twice daily.

- **Power Mushroom and Regeneration:** 1/4 to 1/2 tablet of each formula twice a day.

Vitamins and Herbs Plus Antioxidants—Karen Bentley, DVM

In addition to the individual treatment that your animal may be receiving from a veterinarian, here are a number of natural remedies that can be combined into a helpful supporting program. They include a multi-vitamin mineral supplement, extra vitamin E, the antioxidant CoQ_{10}, kelp, and herbs.

DOSAGE AND OTHER IMPORTANT DETAILS

- **Daily multiple vitamins and minerals:** I recommend combining two excellent products, Mega-C Plus, from Orthomolecular Specialties (408-227-9334), and Maximum Protection Formula, from Dr. Goodpet (800-222-9932). Use full amounts as recommended on each label.

- **Vitamin E:** 100 IU twice a day.

- **CoQ_{10}:** I always recommend coenzyme Q_{10} if you are dealing with a solid tumor. At high doses (300 milligrams), it has anti-tumor effects. In my experience it works better than shark cartilage. Work up to 300 milligrams, divided in to two 150-milligram doses daily. Open the capsules and add the yellow powder into the food.

- **Kelp meal powder:** 1/4 teaspoon daily. Mix into food.

- **Two herbal tinctures:** Hoxsey Red Clover Supreme and Pau d'Arco Inner Bark (alcohol free), both by Gaia Herbs (800-831-7780). The Hoxsey formula is a potent detoxifier and immune system supporter. Pau d'arco is a South American herb well-known for its anticancer properties. Give 5 drops of each tincture two times daily.

Whole-Food Supplements—Joseph Demers, DVM

There are a number of potent products available at health food stores that have substantial anticancer properties. Among them are natural whole-food supplements such as kelp and barley grass. Start with a pinch and increase slowly to the recommended label level over two weeks.

DOSAGE AND OTHER IMPORTANT DETAILS

- **Sea Meal:** This kelp formula made by Solid Gold Health Products for Pets (800-364-4863) nourishes the thyroid gland, which in turn helps to stabilize the endocrine system.

- **Barley Cat:** This product, made by Green Foods Corporation (800-222-3374), contains chlorophyll, antioxidants, amino acids, and enzymes.

My other anticancer recommendations include the following:

- **Essiac tea:** I use an alcohol-extract product from New Action Products (716-873-3738). Add 4 drops to 4 drops of warm water. Stir them together for a moment. That will evaporate the alcohol, and it will taste better. Give directly to the cat twice a day with a dropper.

- **Antioxidant supplements:** Find a good product with vitamins A, C, and E and the mineral selenium. The supplement should at least have these elements. I like to add some of the potent antioxidants such as pycnogenol or grapeseed extract. The daily dosage is a quarter of the recommended human level.

- **Organic flaxseed oil:** This supplement contains important fatty acids believed to be potent nutrients against cancer. Animals don't particularly like the taste of flaxseed oil, so start with 1–2 drops and slowly work up to 1/2 teaspoon daily. Mix into the food.

- **Digestive enzymes:** Cancer patients aren't well animals. They need help with their digestion. Enzymes enable them to extract the maximum nutrition from the food they eat. Follow labels instructions for pet enzyme products.

Multiple Supplement Program—Tejinder Sodhi, DVM

The following supplements are basic elements in a nutritional program to help support animals with cancer. Start low and build up to the recommended levels. The supplements can usually be mixed into the food.

One supplement you may be familiar with as a spice, but not as a nutritional aid, is turmeric. This popular Indian spice contains curcumin, a natural substance with strong anti-inflammatory actions in the body. It also helps boost the immune system. Turmeric is available at most supermarkets, health food stores, and for sure at any Indian store.

Dosage

- **Vitamin C (sodium or calcium ascorbate powder):** Raise slowly to bowel tolerance—that is, to the level where the stool becomes soft (see the discussion on the vitamin C bowel tolerance concept at the beginning of part 2). When you reach this level, reduce the amount slightly. Tolerance varies among individual animals. It is best to give the vitamin C in divided doses throughout the day.

- **Vitamin E:** 100 IU daily.

- **Digestive enzymes:** Use the pet products made from plant sources. Follow label instructions.

- **Coenzyme Q10:** Up to 30 milligrams daily.

- **B complex:** Use a product that has up to 25 milligrams of the major B components.

- **Essiac tea tincture:** 10 drops, two or three times daily.

- **Turmeric:** Mix into the food. Start low and increase gradually up to 1/4 teaspoon.

Pau d'Arco Plus Vitamin C—Maria Glinski, DVM

Pau d'arco is a primary herb I use for all species diagnosed with cancer and immune disorders. It is a powerful immune-boosting agent from Brazil, where it is widely regarded for cancer. I recommend the glycerin-based liquid product from Gaia Herbs (800-831-7780), available at health food stores.

I use the pau d'arco in combination with buffered vitamin C powder (in the form of calcium ascorbate). I have had wonderful results with these two supplements, even for animals given little time to live. Many have gone on to live for years. This is a safe and beneficial long-term program.

DOSAGE
- **Pau d'arco:** 10 drops twice a day.

- **Vitamin C:** Mix with yogurt, which animals will readily eat. Start with 250 milligrams and slowly increase dosage to bowel tolerance (see vitamin C bowel tolerance concept at beginning of part 2).

CHINESE HERBS FOR MAMMARY GLAND TUMORS

Once an animal is diagnosed with breast cancer, the conventional opinion is that it will live about six months if you do not remove the tumor. And if you remove the tumor, they say, the animal will probably be dead because of recurring cancer within two years. In my clinic I recommend surgical removal of the tumor followed by natural remedies on a long-term basis to help prevent recurrences. In my experience I see animals who go on for years and then die of causes other than cancer.

For such tumors, I fortify my supplement program with a traditional Chinese multiple herbal formula called Chih-ko and Curcuma, made by Seven Forests (distributed through I.T.M., at 800-544-7504). The Chinese name for this formula is Xiao Zhong Liu Pian. It is used extensively in China for cancer and comes in the form of an oval tablet.

DOSAGE
- 1/2 tablet twice a day.

Extending Life Naturally—Thomas Van Cise, DVM

In many cases we attain good therapeutic results using a variety of different natural approaches where pet owners chose not to subject their animals to chemotherapy, radiation, or surgery. Frequently tumors go into long-term remission. In general, animals that eventually succumb to the disease live much longer than expected and usually more comfortably, without any of the serious side effects associated with conventional treatment.

The type of natural treatment a holistic practitioner selects depends on the severity of the condition, the tissues involved, and what the owner expects. My approach is basically threefold:

1. Acupuncture, probably ten sessions or more, to stimulate the body to fight off the cancer. This technique also works well to protect animals against side effects from radiation treatments.

2. Shark cartilage. I recommend Benefin shark cartilage made by Lane Laboratories (1-800-LANE-005).

3. Either uña de gato (cat's claw), a South American herb with a powerful effect on tumors, or Dismutase. Choice is often based on the form of the supplement that the owner finds most easy to administer. Dismutase is available in tablet form. The uña de gato that I prefer comes as a liquid.

   Uña de gato is an antioxidant and adaptogen—a substance that helps the body against stress. I have seen tumors disappear over time when this herbal is used. It is also an excellent agent for reducing or eliminating the serious side effects that accompany chemotherapy. I have found Rainforest Bio-Energetics' uña de gato as a reliable herb (available through Van Cise's clinic at 909-737-1242).

   I recall treating two older domestic shorthair cats living in the same household who both had cancer. Tuxedo had a tumor in the wall of the intestine, and Little Mamma had a rapidly growing lymphosarcoma, a mass in the mesentery tissue connecting the intestines. The combination of acupuncture and uña de gato eliminated Tuxedo's tumor, as determined by ultrasound. As for Little Mamma, the treatment arrested the growth of the tumor. The two cats lived on much longer than the veterinary oncologist had predicted.

   Most owners of cancer patients are reluctant to stop therapies that contribute to their pet's recovery. The amount or frequency of dosing uña de gato or other supplements might be lowered once the pet recovers, but it is unlikely that you would want to stop the supplements completely.

   Dismutase is the other supplement I often recommend for strengthening an animal against cancer. The product, made by Bio Vet International (800-788-1084), is a whole-food antioxidant derived from specially grown wheat and soy sprouts. Dismutase helps the body neutralize free radicals, molecular fragments in the body that cause destruction to tissue and accelerate aging and disease. I have found the human version of this product more beneficial than the flavored veterinary tablet.

Dosage

- **Benefin:** 1 gram in either caplet or powder form, preferably on an empty stomach.

- **Uña de gato:** 1/2 dropperful of the liquid three times daily. It works better on an empty stomach.

- **Dismutase:** For most cats, 1 tablet works well. Large cats can take 2 tablets. Preferably give on an empty stomach. Many cats may not eat the tablet, which tastes like dry bread. If this is the case, and you don't want to pill the cat, than grind the tablet into a powder and mix into the food.

Shark Cartilage—Mark Haverkos, DVM

I have been impressed with shark cartilage as part of a cancer treatment program. You have to use it at a very high dose. Originally, when I first tried it some years ago, I didn't see good results. Later I realized the doses were not high enough.

I had an amazing result with a cat who developed abdominal cancer and was treated conventionally to no avail by another veterinarian. We prescribed very high doses of shark cartilage for the animal. A month later the owner brought the cat back to the original vet who had diagnosed the animal. An abdominal tap was performed, and to the amazement of the vet there was no trace of cancer. He performed another tap just to make sure there was no mistake. There was no mistake: the cancer was gone.

Dosage

- 5 to 9 capsules daily of 750-milligram strength.

⚜ Dental Health ⚜

Today's version of *Alice in Wonderland*'s Cheshire cat might not be grinning so widely. Instead it might be grimacing from a toothache. That's because since Alice's day, tooth and gum diseases have become major problems among cats. Nearly half the cat population over the age of three has one kind of dental disorder or another. As many as 85 percent of these cats may suffer from bad gums alone, an incidence similar to that in dogs and people. Oral care, meaning oral hygiene at home and periodic veterinary attention, should be an important part of your overall health care strategy. Some experts, in fact, believe that proper dental care can prolong a pet's life by 20 percent, so this is a subject to take seriously.

Let's take a closer look at the two most common oral problems of cats:

- **Gum disease.** The problem begins with the formation of plaque, a transparent, adhesive fluid composed of bacteria. The bacterial action eats away the supportive gum tissue of the teeth. When plaque is not removed by brushing, cleaning, or an animal eating the right food, mineral salts in the saliva form hard crusts—called "calculus" or "tartar"—over the plaque, which then irritates gum tissue. You see redness and then swelling, the start of gingivitis.

    If neglected, gingivitis turns to periodontitis, a much more serious condition. Animals then develop progressive infection, inflammation, loss of the tiny ligaments that bind the gums to the teeth, bone recession, and loose teeth. Halitosis or bad breath is a primary sign of periodontal disease.

    Chronic oral infections of this nature are not just a problem localized in the mouth. There is further danger of bacteria spreading to other parts and organs of the body, as well as creating a constant burden on the immune system.

- **Cavities.** Cats have been increasingly developing cavities—known also as "feline odontoclastic resorptive lesions" or "neck lesions." The problem was not documented before

1953. The cavities develop at the gum line of the teeth and are usually preceded by tartar buildup. Purebreds, alley cats, and feral cats are all affected.

"These are not really the same kinds of cavities that humans have, but rather a resorption, or breakdown of tooth tissue," says Jan Bellows, DVM, a holistic practitioner in Florida who is one of a handful of certified veterinary dentists. "If untreated, erosion of the tooth will eventually involve the nerve and result in persistent pain. The only real treatment at this point is extraction. Fillings do not work for more than two years because the resorption continues to dissolve the tooth."

At first it was thought that the problem might be related to commercial pet food, but researchers have found that feral cats who do not eat commercial food are also developing this condition. Other possibilities are genetic and environmental.

Some practitioners with a special interest in veterinary dentistry believe that cats who regularly eat a fair amount of raw food have fewer cavities. They think there may be an immune connection.

GENERAL CARE

Dental Dos and Don'ts—Jan Bellows, DVM

(Note: If you have Internet access and desire more information on dental health care for animals, see Dr. Bellows's informative Web site at www.dentalvet.com.)

- **Diet.** In the act of eating prey in the wilds, cats devour fur, hair, and tough elastic tissue that provides a natural brushing effect on their teeth. But our domesticated animals don't eat food with such "built-in" toothbrushes. Often the food is soft. Despite all the benefits of a good home-prepared meal, with raw or cooked meat added, the consistency of the food is overall soft. Cats need something harder included in their diet, something that offers some abrasiveness but doesn't damage gum tissue.

  We often resort to kibble for our animals out of convenience. Ideally the kibble you are feeding your animal should be high quality. Besides convenience, kibble also has a hard consistency that offers a brushing benefit to the teeth before it is mashed into mush. The quality kibble brand I recommend is Cornucopia. It is not a treatment for periodontal disease, but it helps as part of a prevention strategy.

For tartar control and plaque buildup, I recommend a food called t/d—a prescription diet made by Hills and available through veterinarians. The food is designed to provide a brushing effect on the teeth. Nevertheless, it does not take the place of daily brushing.

- **Brushing a must.** Whatever your food choices, you should still brush your animal's teeth if you want to prevent periodontal disease. Brushing is the most important thing you can do for your animal's dental health, and either you do it or face veterinary dental bills later on. If your animal already has gum disease, brushing is critical. Brush every day, just as you do for yourself. Do it twice if possible. Researchers have shown in dogs that if the teeth are cleaned every other day, the preventive effect still works. If you do it less often, forget it. You might as well not bother. It involves an effort, and many of my clients accept the daily brushing because I make a major issue of it.

- **Use a natural, soft-bristled brush.** Veterinarians and pet stores sell special oral care products. St. Jon's makes a number of good products. You can also purchase "natural" toothpaste at the health food store. Some of the brands I like are Nature's Gate (cherry gel), Peelu, and Dessert Essence. If the cat doesn't like the taste, try dipping the brush first in a can of tuna in water and allow the bristles to sop up some of the tuna juice.

- **How to brush.** When you do this for the first time, approach your cat gently. If you can start the brushing habit when your cat is young, it's quite easy, but even older pets will accept the process. Try to work the bristles of the brush under the gums. Place the bristles at the gum margin of the teeth. Move the brush in a circular or back-and-forth motion. Gently press the bristle ends into the area around the base of the tooth as well as into the space between the teeth. You can generally cover three or four teeth at a time. Ten strokes should be completed at each location. This is what it takes to clear out the daily accumulation of plaque. If not cleared, it builds up underneath the gums and leads to inflammation, gingivitis, and eventually periodontal disease. The upper teeth attract the most plaque, so spend the most time there.

- **For noncooperative animals.** If your cat isn't receptive to brushing no matter what, use a washcloth or piece of gauze to wipe the teeth, front and back. Gently rub the teeth clean around the gum line. With luck you can graduate to a tooth-brush, which is preferable. That's what it takes to get under the gum line.

- **If the gums bleed when brushed.** See your veterinarian.

- **Examine your animal's teeth and gums monthly.** Most cats don't mind if you peek inside their mouths. Look for inflammation (redness), swelling, and broken teeth. A good place to search for inflammation is in the back of the mouth, where the upper fourth premolar teeth meet the gum tissue. This site is where the salivary glands secrete into the mouth. The fourth premolars are the fourth tooth back on each side from the canine, the so-called fang tooth or eyetooth. Your examination should include the entire face. One side should look the same as the other, with no abnormal swellings. When looking at the head, feel the glands under your pet's neck. Both should be the same size. If one is swollen, that could indicate an abscess or infection in the mouth. Be alert for any swelling under the eye. That may be another sign of an abscess.

- **Smell your pet's breath.** If it smells very bad, that's a sign of gum disease or digestive problems. See your veterinarian.

- **A regular dental checkup by your veterinarian is advisable.** Gingivitis can usually be reversed with a thorough cleaning by a veterinarian while the animal is anesthetized. If treated early, the gums can return to normal appearance and function. If left untreated, periodontitis results. If you need a specialist, contact the American Veterinary Dental Society (800-332-AVDS).

- **Tooth pain.** Cloves are a good stopgap measure for relief until you can see a veterinarian. Cloves contain analgesic properties. Apply the ground clove directly to the affected area.

- **Vitamin C and coenzyme Q_{10} to fight gum disease.** In humans, a low level of vitamin C in the tissues is associated with a predisposition to periodontal disease. Use vitamin C in the form of sodium ascorbate crystals mixed in the food. The vitamin decreases pain, builds up the immune system against infections, and helps to fortify connective tissue and the tiny ligaments binding tooth to gum. Coenzyme Q_{10} is a fat-soluble vitamin and antioxidant that decreases inflammation, swelling, and pocket depths. The mouth must be cleaned first professionally in order for this nutrient to have a pronounced impact.

Dosage

- **Vitamin C:** Start with 100 milligrams twice a day, then increase the daily dose by 250 milligrams each week, until bowel tolerance is reached (see description of vitamin C bowel tolerance concept at the beginning of part 2).

- **Coenzyme Q_{10}:** 10 milligrams twice daily

Supplement for Better Oral Health—Ron Carsten, DVM

If you have a cat with gum and tooth problems, a good general nutritional supplement to specifically benefit the mouth is Biodent. This human product, made by Standard Process (800-848-5061), can be ordered for you by your veterinarian. It contains bone meal, carrot powder, spleen, and other nutrients that create a healthier chemistry in the tissue of the mouth. The product helps contain inflammation, while supporting any veterinary treatment that is being given.

Biodent can help reverse deficiencies that have often existed for years. It takes time to work, so be patient. Keep the mouth clean. Brush the teeth on a daily basis if possible, and keep building up the tissue with these nutrients. And remember that when you feed animals better food, including some raw meat and vegetables, they tend not to develop a lot of the typical oral conditions.

Dosage
- 1 tablet twice a day.

Dentifrice to Counteract Plaque—Alfred Plechner, DVM

Polish your cat's teeth and gums regularly with Pearl Drops, a dentifrice available in drugstores. This does a good job to clean the mouth and counteract plaque formation. Apply the drops with gauze or a washcloth.

If you are interested in performing a more rigorous form of oral housekeeping, ask your veterinarian to show you how to use a dental scaler on your animal. Scaling the teeth once a month is a good way to prevent plaque buildup.

Calendula for General Gum Care—Thomas Van Cise, DVM

To help prevent gum disease, apply Calendula, a homeopathic remedy. Purchase a bottle of the mother tincture in a homeopathic pharmacy or health food store. Put 6 drops in 1 ounce of distilled water. Brush with this solution on a daily basis, if possible. If there is any inflammation, brushing may irritate the gums. In that case, use a cotton swab padded with extra cotton (from a cotton ball) so that it soaks up the liquid. Cover both the outside and inside of the gums with the Calendula.

Special Supplement "Chews"—Jean Hofve, DVM

CET Forte Chews, made by VRX Pharmaceuticals (800-969-7387) and sold through veterinarians, is a helpful preventive supplement. These freeze-dried nuggets are shaped somewhat like packing peanuts. They give teeth and gums a good workout and cleaning and definitely contribute to a healthy mouth. The individual pieces are impregnated with enzymes to synergize with natural enzymes in the mouth. They also contain protein and antioxidants. Most cats will eat them readily.

You have to start with clean teeth. I have not found that the supplement removes any significant amount of tartar even though the manufacturer claims it will. My advice is to start using it after a dental cleaning and give it at least every other day. It takes forty-eight hours for tartar to harden. The product is relatively expensive, but you may save money in the long run on dental bills, not to mention the trauma and anesthetic risks to your cat that are involved in dental treatments.

I believe that much of the tooth problem in cats has a genetic background. I see it more in certain breeds, and certain colors, and other veterinarians have said the same thing. Redheaded cats have more gingivitis than other cats. Purebreds are clearly more at risk for dental problems. Among them, Abyssinians and Persians seem to have more problems, Maine Coons less. If you see an Abyssinian over the age of four with any teeth, that's a pretty hardy cat. They tend to lose all their teeth and have weak immunity. You have to monitor Abyssinians very closely. The mouth is the first thing to go; it is the gateway to the respiratory and digestive systems. When the immune system is weak, you see lots of tartar building up, with gingivitis and inflammation. Cats with feline leukemia and feline AIDS frequently have bad mouths.

INFLAMED GUMS

Echinacea-Goldenseal—Karen Bentley, DVM

For red, inflamed gums, the topical application of an herbal combination called Echinacea-Goldenseal Supreme, by Gaia Herbs (800-831-7780), can help to make a cat's mouth more comfortable. The liquid product is available in many health food stores.

This condition usually reflects an underlying weakness of the immune system. Rounds of antibiotics that are often prescribed do not address the cause of the problem and in many cases lead to new symptoms elsewhere, such as intestinal upset. It is important to build up an animal's immune system whenever you see gum disorders.

DOSAGE
- Saturate a Q-tip with the liquid. Run it along the gum line once a day. If the condition is severe, do it twice a day.

CAVITIES
(FELINE ODONTOCLASTIC RESORPTIVE LESIONS)

Vitamin C a Powerful Preventive—Jan Bellows, DVM

To help prevent the problem I recommend two things:

1. **Regular brushing of the teeth** (see how to brush in Bellows's foregoing commentary). Until we know what precisely causes the cavities, we can't say that brushing will totally eliminate the problem. But we know that brushing helps because it cuts down the plaque.

2. **Vitamin C.** In hundreds of cases I have observed that vitamin C has a powerful preventive effect against cat cavities. I simply don't see cavities when people start their young animals on vitamin C. If a cat owner brings in a cat with a cavity, we start vitamin C right away, and usually there are no recurrences. The form of vitamin C I recommend is sodium ascorbate crystals, mixed into the food.

DOSAGE

- Start at 100 milligrams twice daily and then increase the dose slowly each week. For severe cases I may go up to 1,000 milligrams. Most cats do well on 250 milligrams twice daily.

Vitamin C and CoQ$_{10}$—Carvel Tiekert, DVM

Vitamin C and coenzyme Q$_{10}$ help prevent this deterioration. However, a number of veterinarians believe that starting kittens on raw meat may be the most important preventive measure you can take.

If the cat is already affected, supplements help slow down the deterioration, but the animal will probably require monitoring or treatment on a regular basis. We can help these cats, but I don't think we cure them. Individualized treatment with a veterinarian homeopath may also be of help.

DOSAGE

- **Vitamin C:** 250 to 500 milligrams a day, in the form of nonacidic crystals (sodium or calcium ascorbate). Mix into the food.

- **CoQ$_{10}$:** 10 milligrams daily.

Barnyard Cats Don't Get Cavities—Roger DeHaan, DVM

When I attended veterinary school more than thirty years ago, a professor told us that cats didn't get cavities. Now they do, and the problem is rampant. Some cats have up to a couple of dozen of them. The gums become red and inflamed because of the food that catches in there. You can clean up the teeth and the condition comes right back.

"Barnyard cats eating live food do not get dental cavities," a lecturer once said at a dental course I took. "Only cats on commercial cat foods get them." Barnyard cats, of course, are living off their prey, the raw food they capture.

No exact cause of the cavities has been found by researchers. Some say it is the chemical contents of common tap water. Others say it is the food. What we do know for sure is that most animals out on their own don't get it. The modern domesticated cat does. So do alley cats and feral cats.

My conclusion is that this is an environmental/nutritional issue of some kind. Alley and feral cats are still eating a large degree of "junk" food that they scavenge. The food is unbalanced and often contaminated. They are nutritionally and immunologically depleted also. The food they eat is is raised on the same depleted soil as the commercial food eaten by companion cats.

My suggestion is to feed a more natural diet. Be sure to supplement. Modern food just doesn't have it anymore. I suggest a whole-food supplement such as Missing Link, made by Designing Health, Inc. (800-774-7387), and extra vitamin C. And give animals filtered or purified water, if possible. You cannot reverse this problem once it occurs. Thereafter you are dealing with dental care. But you can slow down future reabsorption. Prevention is the best solution while you have a healthy cat. That means feeding a healthier diet along with a whole-food supplement.

Cats may not like having their teeth brushed. So a good alternative is to use a fifty-fifty combination of baking soda and hydrogen peroxide on a Q-tip to rub the teeth along the gum. The baking soda alkalizes the acid-loving bacteria, and the hydrogen peroxide oxidizes them. The effect is a double-barrel zapping of bacteria. Such routine home care will not reverse the condition. The holes are still there under the gum and will collect bacteria. But you can slow down the progress and may even stop further cavities. You must do it daily or at least every other day. Anything less probably won't do any good.

DOSAGE
- **Missing Link:** Follow label instructions.

- **Vitamin C:** 100 to 250 milligrams daily.

⚓ Diabetes ⚓

Diabetes, or high blood sugar, is a metabolic disorder that affects many older, obese cats. Similar to adult onset diabetes in humans, feline diabetes results when the aging feline pancreas no longer produces enough insulin (the vital hormone that allows blood sugar to be transported into cells and burned for energy) or the cells of the body lose their ability to use it properly.

Signs of diabetes in cats are unquenchable thirst, increased urination, and a ravenous appetite, many times accompanied by weight loss. If your cat develops these signs, see a veterinarian immediately. Creating an effective management program for a diabetic cat requires professional experience, whether you choose a conventional or holistic approach. Unless the condition is brought under control, it can cause vomiting, loss of appetite, weakness, dehydration, poor skin and hair coat, liver disease, many different metabolic disturbances, and ultimately death.

Holistic veterinarians believe that cats fed a wholesome, species-appropriate diet from kittenhood are much less likely to develop diabetes. They successfully treat many diabetic animals with a natural diet and supplements alone, without insulin. Conventionally, diabetes is managed through prescription-type diets and insulin medication, either injected or taken orally.

Diet, Enzymes, and Supplements—Roger DeHaan, DVM
One of the keys to success in dealing with diabetes is to feed your animal a "whole natural food" diet and stick to it. I have seen many

cats over the years who did not respond to insulin because they were eating some junky cat food. So, no junk and no snacks. That alone may be 50 percent of the solution.

There is evidence that diabetes is in part a problem of pancreatic insufficiency and of breaking down foods. For this reason, the use of digestive enzymes is helpful to enable animals to process food more effectively. Use any of the good products for animals, such as Florazyme, from Pet's Friend (800-868-1009), or Feline Digestive Enzymes, from Dr. Goodpet (800-222-9932). Follow label instructions.

I have had good results over the years using a combination of chromium, vitamin E, and selenium. Each of these elements has proven benefits against diabetes. Chromium stimulates insulin activity. Insulin must first combine with chromium in order to effectively open the tissues to glucose and the production of energy. Experiments show that insulin is virtually powerless without adequate chromium to create energy. Processed food is typically deficient in chromium. Studies also show that chromium supplementation reduces blood sugar. Vitamin E and selenium are important antioxidants that can help protect the blood vessels and other tissue from accelerated oxidative damage caused by high blood sugar levels.

Another useful mineral nutrient is vanadium in the form of vanadium sulfate. This trace mineral can mimic the effects of insulin or increase its efficiency in the body, thus reducing both blood sugar and insulin levels. A word of caution, however. When using chromium or vanadium supplements, be sure to monitor the blood sugar level regularly. You don't want to cause such a sharp drop that you create a hypoglycemic effect—that is, low blood sugar.

DOSAGE
- **Vitamin E:** 30 IU.

- **Chelated chromium:** 30 micrograms.

- **Chelated selenium:** 30 micrograms.

- **Vanadium sulfate:** 5 micrograms daily or 10 micrograms every other day.

Feed Homemade Meals—Jean Hofve, DVM

Most veterinarians put diabetic animals on w/d, a high-fiber dry food made by Science Diet. This is a "fat cat" diet. It has a lot of fiber in it, and the concept is that the fiber slows the digestive process and will act to keep the blood glucose level steadier over time. However, there has never been any scientific proof that this is helpful.

You want diabetics to eat and be happy. Feed them healthful foods they enjoy. Food should be readily available. When diabetic animals need food, they really need it. I don't recommend any currently available commercial food as even remotely good for diabetic cats, although a high-quality dry food left out may be useful as a backup in emergencies (refer to dry food recommendations in chapter 5).

Cats, diabetics or otherwise, need a high-protein, high-fat, and low-carbohydrate diet. This is the closest to the fresh prey they were designed by nature to eat. Commercial dry foods are high in carbohydrates, mainly in the form of cereal grains, for which cats have no dietary requirement and cannot adequately digest.

Consider preparing food at home that consists of approximately 60 percent protein (meat) and 30 percent fat. Add bone meal as a good source of calcium, plus a vitamin and mineral supplement (see Hofve's "Easy Cat Recipe" in chapter 6). It's not that hard to do. If you can't do this, at least add some fresh meat daily to a very good-quality commercial diet.

In diagnosed cases, I suggest adding flaxseed oil, a source of omega-3 fatty acids that have antioxidant, anti-inflammatory benefits and are great for the flaky skin and dry coat problems common in diabetic cats. This can be substituted for part of the fat content of the daily diet. Some cats may not like the taste. I personally find Barlean's organic oil (800-445-3529) to be the most palatable. Start with a very small amount and increase gradually. If the cat won't "volunteer" to eat it in the food, then ask your veterinarian for a 3-cc syringe and squirt the oil directly into the mouth. An alternative is to use a good daily pet supplement that includes flaxseed oil or ground flaxseed and is more palatable, such as Missing Link, made by Designing Health, Inc. (800-774-7387).

Gamma linoleic acid (GLA) is reported to prevent or reduce diabetic neuropathy, a degenerative change in the nerves, usually seen in the hind legs of diabetic cats. Evening primrose oil is a good source of GLA.

I also use Cataplex GTF, which contains chromium, and Diaplex, with pancreatic glandular extract, liver support, and digestive enzymes. These products are made by Standard Process (800-848-5061), which are sold through health professionals and veterinarians and need to be tailored individually to the specific cat.

DOSAGE
- **Flaxseed oil:** 1/4 to 1/2 teaspoon.

- **Evening primrose oil:** 1/4 teaspoon.

⚜ Diarrhea ⚜

See Digestive Disorders.

⚜ Digestive Disorders ⚜

The section is divided into the following conditions, some of which have similar causes: constipation, diarrhea and vomiting, inflammatory bowel disease, digestive enzyme deficiency, and gas.

CONSTIPATION

Constipation is common among cats, particularly older animals. The colon doesn't have the oomph it had in younger days to move fecal matter out of the body. Hairballs can cause the problem at any age (see hairballs).

Limit Food Access and No Dry Food—Michele Yasson, DVM

There are a few things you can do to remedy this problem:

- **Feed only once or twice a day.** Carnivores are meant to have big bundles of food move through their digestive tracts. A mouse at a time, for a cat. Nibbling all day doesn't give a good push through to the other end; it is just a minor stimulation. A small amount of stool reaches the hind end and just sits there. But when a large bolus of stool comes through, then there is stimulus to go.

- **No dry food.** Cats are a desert species and become dehydrated on dry food. I have treated many cats who were diagnosed by other veterinarians with kidney failure when what they really had was dehydration caused by dry food. I switched them to canned food or, better yet, home-prepared food, and they start showing much better kidney function and better bowel movement. The more lubricated the plumbing, the better things move through.

- **Use a product called Capra Mineral Whey** (made by Mt. Capra Cheese, 800-574-1961), a unique and easily absorbed natural supplement for humans in powder form derived from goat's milk. Whey is a natural tonic for the intestines and is extremely useful for constipation cases. I find it is almost as good as the heavy-duty conventional drugs. It is a "whole food," so an animal can be on it indefinitely. It also provides a rich source of biologically active minerals. Most cats like the taste.

  DOSAGE
  - One-quarter of the human dose. Mix into the food.

Metamucil and Cow's Milk for Relief—Lynne Friday, DVM

I see a lot of constipation in overweight and overfed cats. A low thyroid can also lead to constipation because the body's mechanisms move sluggishly, including the bowels. If you notice your cat is constipated, see a vet. The problem may be megacolon and require treatment. Otherwise, here are some approaches that will help keep them loose if they have a tendency to constipation:

- Metamucil.
- Cow's milk (give them 1 tablespoon).
- Green beans baby food.

If you need to take bolder action, a coffee enema is very effective. This method promotes detoxification of tissues and blood, and the elimination of toxic bile, by stimulating enzyme systems in the gut wall and liver. Use 1 tablespoon of instant coffee for each cup of warm water. A cat will take a pint of liquid.

Suck up the mix in a rubber ear bulb syringe that you would use to flush out the ears. Put some Vaseline or vegetable oil on the stem of the syringe to help it go in smoothly. Insert it into the animal's rectum and gently flush out the colon. Don't instill all the liquid at one time. Instill a portion of the liquid, then let the animal walk around. Then repeat. The enema process can be done over a half hour.

Feeding animals too many bones can also contribute to constipation. Particularly troublesome are pork bones, which are brittle and break up easily. They can create a cementlike impaction in the colon and actually rip the intestinal walls as they come out. I have had to knock out some animals and pull out the pieces. By then the rectum is bleeding badly.

Slippery Elm—Norman C. Ralston, DVM

You can counteract constipation by using the herb slippery elm in powder form, available at health food stores. You should see improved bowel function in a day or two.

DOSAGE
- 1 teaspoon mixed into the food.

Acupuncture—Nancy Scanlan, DVM

Acupuncture works well for extreme cases where cats haven't gone for days and days. Constipation is a frequent problem among Manx cats, who have an abnormality of the nervous system in the hindquarter that affects intestinal function. Usually these animals require ongoing treatment, which may be as often as once a week or just once or twice a year. There are simple acupressure techniques that a knowledgeable veterinarian can teach to pet owners to help promote evacuation.

GRASS-EATING CATS—NORMAN C. RALSTON, DVM

Cats often like to chomp on grass. It gives them fiber and helps with proper elimination. If you have an indoor cat, try this approach that was told to me by a client who lives on the twelfth floor of an apartment building. She raises wheatgrass in the window, and whenever the cat has the urge, it jumps onto the ledge and has a healthy nibble.

DIARRHEA AND VOMITING
(See also "Inflammatory Bowel Disease" and
"Food Allergies")

There are two kinds of diarrhea: acute or chronic. The acute form often relates to "garbage gut." Your animal has eaten something that has upset the stomach. If this continues longer than a day, see your veterinarian for an examination and fecal test, particularly if the animal is an outdoor type.

A sudden diet change can bring on diarrhea. Always make your switches slowly, over a period of ten days or more.

In any case of a persistent problem, whatever the cause, see a veterinarian. The problem often relates to inflammatory bowel disease and food allergies and can be caused or triggered by vaccinations. Many cases can be resolved with a homemade diet without chemical additives or special limited antigen diets (see the section on food allergies) sold by veterinarians.

Parasites such as *Giardia* (protozoa) can cause a horrendous watery and smelly diarrhea and can be picked up by drinking contaminated water. *Giardia* is prevalent in water coming out of the Rockies.

Many holistic veterinarians recommend probiotics for diarrhea. Probiotics are nutritional supplements, available at all health food stores, that contain billions of beneficial bacteria, such as *Lactobacillus acidophilus* and *Bifidobacterium bifidum*. Many strains of beneficial bacteria are normally present in the gut and perform numerous functions critical to health, including the production of important enzymes, containment of pathological microorganisms, and protection against the formation of cancerous substances. Frequently animals become depleted as a result of taking medications and antibiotics. Antibiotics not only destroy pathogenic bacteria, but also devastate the population of good bacteria. The loss of these beneficial microorganisms can cause vomiting, diarrhea, liver problems, immune imbalances, and allergies.

Using Probiotics—Ron Carsten, DVM

Antibiotics are infamous for disrupting the normal, essential digestive bacteria. Dogs seem to develop more problems from antibiotics than do cats. Cats appear to be fairly resistant. Nevertheless, disturbances in the digestive tract can and do happen as a result.

To avoid the problems frequently associated with antibiotics and either maintain or restore the beneficial bacteria population in the gut, start giving the probiotic concurrently with any antibiotic treatment your veterinarian has prescribed. Continue for at least two weeks or more after the antibiotics are completed.

When I treat an animal with a history of multiple antibiotic treatments and digestive problems, I routinely prescribe a probiotic supplement. Quite often I see a major improvement that I relate to the restoration of a bacterial balance. These cases frequently involve cats who had antibiotic courses as kittens and subsequently developed inefficient or compromised digestive systems. I recommend using the probiotic for at least one month in such cases and ideally for two or three months to fully reestablish the beneficial bacterial colony in the gut.

Probiotics come in different forms—usually as liquids or capsules.

DOSAGE
- There is no exact science for dosing. In general, give your cat the equivalent of about 3 to 6 billion microorganisms twice a day. Monitor your animal closely, and reduce the dose or discontinue the product if problems arise. There may be some individual variation in response. Some patients may be unable to accept a higher dose. This is likely owing to the overall health and condition of the digestive tract. A problem could indicate the presence of other digestive disorders that need to

be identified by a veterinarian. It is a good idea to obtain a stool evaluation to determine bacterial status. A reevaluation of the stool after the probiotic has been given for some time is also useful to assess whether bacterial balance has improved.

The "Fast" Solution—Charles Loops, DVM

The large majority of diarrhea and vomiting situations resolve in twenty-four hours if you fast the animal. If the problem is diarrhea, provide only liquid for the twenty-four hours. If the animal is vomiting, do not give any food or liquid.

Be observant. If the diarrhea or vomiting are severe and continuing, see a veterinarian.

Baby Food After the Fast—Jean Hofve, DVM

The simplest solution for acute diarrhea is to withhold food for about twenty-four hours and then start the animal back on something bland, such as baby food. Any of the baby meat foods is a wonderful remedy for initiating the eating process after the fast. Cats will eat it when they are too sick to eat anything else. But read the label. The product cannot have onion powder—this is toxic to cats. It will cause anemia if you feed enough of it. Baby food is not balanced and should be relied upon not for long-term use, but merely as a transition to regular food.

Fasting Plus Probiotics Plus Clay—Donna Starita Mehan, DVM

As a general rule, the basic recommendation is to fast the animal for a day. Water is okay, but let the digestive tract have a rest.

Provide your animal with a probiotic supplement. Also, utilize a good bentonite clay product, usually available at health food stores. This mineral powder swells up, slows down the bowels, and acts as an intestinal broom, sweeping away toxins.

DOSAGE
- 1/4 teaspoon twice daily. Mix the powder into a little yogurt or broth.

Homeopathics Plus Probiotics—Carvel Tiekert, DVM

For the uncomplicated, now-and-then variety of diarrhea, I recommend any of the widely available homeopathic combination remedies for diarrhea along with a probiotic supplement.

Slippery Elm, Nux Vomica, and Clay—Roger DeHaan, DVM

Slippery elm is a nutritive herb that heals, soothes, and nourishes the inflamed digestive tract. I usually recommend Nux vomica, a homeopathic remedy, along with it. Nux vomica counteracts nausea, irritation, and chemical upset in the stomach and upper intestine.

About 50 percent of cats I treat who vomit daily or several times a week respond immediately to this combination. Within a day or two many others are substantially improved.

An alternative approach is using a third each of slippery elm, aloe vera gel, and powdered bentonite clay, all available in health food stores. The clay has the unique property of pulling out toxins from the intestinal tract. Usually where there is inflammation there are poisons. Bentonite is also a rich source of trace minerals.

Often the problems of diarrhea and vomiting are caused by wrong diet, chemical sensitivities, or reactions to vaccinations. If the remedies don't work, consult with a holistic veterinarian.

DOSAGE

- **Slippery elm:** 1 capsule twice a day. Mix in warm water or chicken broth. Give at time of feeding.

- **Nux vomica 30X:** Twice daily. If a severe episode is occurring, give hourly for four hours, and then three or four times a day as needed. Don't give with food.

- **Bentonite clay:** 1/2 teaspoon of powder mixed in food.

Nux Vomica for Upsets, Irregularity—Maria Glinski, DVM

Nux vomica is a useful homeopathic remedy for any gastrointestinal tract imbalance, particularly for cats who have off-and-on diarrhea or constipation. The remedy works quickly, restoring balance and normal motility to the gut.

Dosage
- **Nux vomica 30C:** 1 or 2 drops twice a day for three days.

Pectin for Diarrhea—Nancy Scanlan, DVM

For both acute and chronic diarrhea, mix pectin into the animal's food. Pectin is a natural form of fiber found in all plant cell walls and in the skin and rind of fruits and vegetables. It has a gel-forming property that acts effectively to bind a loose bowel. It is important to mix it into the food *before feeding*, so it absorbs moisture. If you just sprinkle it on top, it will form a hard rock in the stomach and animals will throw it up. Pectin supplements are available at health food stores.

Dosage
- 1/8 teaspoon.

Chinese Curing Pills Plus Pepto-Bismol—Jody Kincaid, DVM

A Chinese herbal formula appropriately called Curing Pills is a useful natural remedy for an uncomplicated upset stomach or vomiting. I recommend it along with Pepto-Bismol, which will coat and soothe the stomach lining. Curing Pills is a human product and comes in the form of tiny, BB-size pills. It is available in health food stores or Chinese pharmacies.

- **Curing Pills:** 1 pill three times a day.

- **Pepto-Bismol:** 1/2 teaspoon. If the stomach seems really upset, administer every two hours. If the problem persists for more than a day, or a more serious condition is involved, see a veterinarian.

INFLAMMATORY BOWEL DISEASE

Chronic episodes of vomiting and diarrhea can be a sign of inflammatory bowel disease (IBD), also known as irritable bowel syndrome. This common problem requires professional attention because it can create dehydration and become life-threatening. Vomiting and diarrhea have many causes, such as food, allergies, bacteria, or parasites. IBD is another cause, particularly in middle-aged or older cats. Experts say that abnormal immune cell responses are believed to be involved.

A medication called metronidazole is highly effective in rapidly clearing up the condition if it is due to a bacterial overload. When bacteria or parasites are not involved, the cause is probably allergic in nature, creating irritation, inflammation, and turmoil in the stomach or intestines and frequently skin allergies as well. Steroids are frequently used to reduce inflammation, and, if necessary, powerful immunosuppressive drugs.

The Antioxidant Approach—Wendell Belfield, DVM

I have had nearly total success—when no bacteria or parasites are involved—with an antioxidant formula I developed called Vital Liquid, available through Orthomolecular Specialties (408-227-9334). The formula contains vitamins A and E, and selenium and helps keep oxidative damage under control in the bowel. Patients usually respond to this supplement within a week. Diarrhea and vomiting stop.

Some animals need to be maintained permanently on the supplement. Others can come off of it and are fine. Stress and allergies can trigger recurrences. Should that occur, return to the initial therapeutic dosage.

I don't recommend vitamin C for irritable bowel patients because they tend to have a low threshold or tolerance for the vitamin. Always feed your animal high-quality food, particularly those with this condition.

Dosage
• Follow label instructions.

The Food Allergy Connection—Alfred Plechner, DVM

This problem often has to do with food allergies and abnormal activity of antibodies in the mucous membrane of the intestinal tract, a result of imbalances in the endocrine-immune systems (see Plechner's discussion on this problem in the food allergy section and in chapter 15).

DIGESTIVE ENZYME DEFICIENCY

You are what you digest. The same is true for your pets. That's why many veterinarians and pet nutrition experts increasingly recommend digestive enzyme supplements. Digestive enzymes are produced in the pancreas and salivary glands and help break down the protein, carbohydrate, and fat components of food for use by the body. As animals age, the production of these enzymes often slows down. Supplements are particularly beneficial to aging animals with slumping enzyme production. Deficiencies can also be genetically related, and symptoms will show up among kittens.

Research shows a strong connection between deficiencies and diseases—both acute and chronic. Common signs of deficiencies are voluminous stool, often with undigested fat clearly visible, and animals who are overtly underweight despite big appetites.

Many holistic veterinarians use enzyme supplements as a primary tool in dealing with many different problems. In some cases they recommend enzymes alone, while in many others it is one part of a multiple-remedy approach. Improved hair coat and skin, increased vigor, a reduction in allergic problems, and maintenance of good body weight are typical benefits of supplementation. Many animals also become more resistant to disease and infections when supplemented. Veterinarians say that enzymes may also aid older animals suffering from joint ailments. By enhancing digestion and absorption of nutrients, including antioxidants and the mineral magnesium, the body is better able to counteract harmful degenerative processes.

Digestive enzyme formulas contain the individual enzyme components that break down different kinds of food. Protease is the enzyme that breaks down protein; amylase works on carbohydrate; and lipase is the fat-breaking enzyme. Veterinarians advise that it is important to use supplements with a balanced formula of enzymes.

Over the years, plant-based supplements have been developed from *Aspergillis oryzae* (a fungus) that have been found to be effective, and much less expensive, than prescription enzyme products derived from animals. Pet enzyme supplements are widely available in health food stores and pet stores.

Enzymes to Combat Malabsorption—Alfred Plechner, DVM

Malabsorption, the inability to properly absorb nutrients from food, is a major problem that isn't talked about much. I find a huge percentage of my patients cannot digest food properly. The problem may be a lack of digestive enzymes, and in particular, trypsin.

Trypsin is a major pancreatic digestive enzyme that contributes to the breakdown of protein, fats, and carbohydrates. In my practice I routinely test animals for trypsin. Over the years I have determined that nearly a quarter of them have small or moderate trypsin deficiencies.

The impact of deficiency can show up early in kittens, as soon as they start eating solid food. They may grow at a slower pace or not reach full size. The signs could also possibly take several years to show. Often there is an allergiclike dermatitis, hair loss, poor hair coat, and red, scaly itchy skin that an animal gnaws on constantly. You may see large, multiple stools, often with undigested fat clearly visible.

Animals with an enzyme deficiency are often thought to be thin despite a ravenous appetite. Not so in every case. Sometimes the deficiency may contribute to obesity. Many commercial foods have poor-quality, adulterated sources of protein that are hard to break down. The carbohydrates may be easier to break down. So an animal eating voluminous amounts of food in order to get more nutrition will take in more—and absorb more—carbohydrates. This translates to more calories and may result in weight gain.

The causes for trypsin deficiency are basically twofold:

1. **Genetic.** When I first became interested in this problem, I traced a deficiency through generations of Abbysinians and Persians. One generation passed it along to the next. Now I find it in virtually all breeds, pure and mixed. The problem is a result of a widespread hormonal-immune disorder due to contemporary breeding practices (see chapter 15 for more information on this problem).

2. **Acquired.** Viral and bacterial infection, or any insult to the pancreas, such as a food allergy or reaction to a toxin and chemical, can affect trypsin production. The aging process also slows down the pancreas and often interferes with enzyme activity. I find this problem present now in practically all breeds, regardless of age.

Even if there is no deficiency, or if there is only a mild one, many animals simply do not have the digestive juices to break down the highly concentrated and processed food they are fed. The result is malabsorption of food and, to some degree, food allergies (see section on food allergies).

One sign of malabsorption is an animal eating nonfood items. You would be surprised at some of the things that are eaten. Plastic. Socks. Panty hose. Thread. String. Paper. This unnatural craving is called "pica." In my opinion it is caused by a number of things, such as an enzyme deficiency in which an animal can't fulfill its nutritional needs; a mineral deficiency—that is, not enough trace minerals in the diet; and food sensitivities that aggravate the gut and interfere with normal absorption.

The solution for these kinds of problems is often fairly simple—the addition of a good digestive enzyme supplement mixed into the food. The product I use is Power for Life, made by Terra Oceana (805-563-2634), which contains not only enzymes, but a wide range of nutrients, trace minerals, and whole-food factors.

DOSAGE
• Follow label instructions.

Boost Digestion with Enzymes—Allen M. Schoen, DVM

Prozyme (800-522-5537) is an excellent product that I have used for years. It works well for animals with poor absorption, belching, and gas and for geriatric animals who do not have the same level and efficiency of digestive enzymes as when they were younger.

GAS

Yes, it's not just a dog (or people) thing. There are plenty of gassy cats.

Better Diet Plus Enzymes—Carvel Tiekert, DVM

Experiment with the diet. Often I find the problem disappears when you introduce a higher-quality diet, particularly if the cat will eat some raw food.

Plant-based digestive enzymes, which are widely available for pets, resolve the problem in most cases. I have found them generally effective for animals with gas who are already on a good diet, as well as those on the cheaper foods that cause considerable gas. If plant-based enzymes don't work, try pancreatic extracts (animal-based products) before giving up on enzymes.

Ginger—Lynne Friday, DVM
Grate a tiny bit of ginger and add it to the food. The cat may or may not eat it. It's worth a try

---

⚚ Drug Side Effects ⚚

See Poisoning, Drug Side Effects, and Toxicity

⚚ Ear Problems ⚚

Ear problems are not as common in cats as in dogs, but they nevertheless happen, and felines are susceptible to ear mite infestations.

The Stress and Food Connection—Paul McCutcheon, DVM
You have to ask yourself why your cat continually scratches its ears. You can use as much medication as you can stick down the ear canal, but that won't resolve the initiating reason. Topical steroids may clear up the problem temporarily, but symptoms may return and become chronic. Unless there are mites involved (and you deal with that accordingly), the problem is usually caused by a drop in the local immunity. Steroids won't help that. You need to look at potential stress factors (see McCutcheon's entry under stress) or consider offending substances in the pet's diet or environment. Look for the reasons and do not just treat the symptoms.

A Sign of Internal Problems—Roger DeHaan, DVM

Chronic ear problems, when both ears are involved, indicate allergies, an ailing liver or kidneys, or some other internal disorder. Skin is like a third kidney, an organ of elimination, an outlet for toxins. And the ears are part of the skin. When you see problems there over and over, you have to look inside and treat the whole animal. You can run blood tests all day and they may come up normal. Liver and kidney trouble doesn't show up until the organs are 75 percent compromised. For continual ear problems, I recommend a holistic veterinarian who can dig down into the cause.

One basic thing you can do on your own is to change the diet to more wholesome, natural food.

MITES

Mites are tiny parasites that are found throughout the animal kingdom, living on rodents, dogs, and wild and domestic cats. The favorite food of these creatures, it turns out, is ear wax. The presence of mites is usually confirmed by microscopic identification, but if you see a cat that is scratching its ears constantly and you see a deposit inside the ears that looks like dried coffee grinds, then you have a good reason to suspect a mite infestation. If untreated, the problem can lead to bacterial and fungal infections or pus and spread to the inner ear and cause deafness.

This problem should be treated by a veterinarian, certainly if there is any sign of pus. If you do try the natural remedies suggested here and they don't work, don't waste time in seeing a vet. Don't go to your local pet store and buy their ear mite fixer. It will make a mess and generally won't work. The cat will become very upset with you...and still have the mites. Just let your veterinarian treat it with medication. It works.

Generally, healthy animals have fewer problems with ear mites.

Olive Oil and Yellow Dock—William Pollak, DVM

Step 1: Mix 1/2 ounce of olive oil and 400 IU of vitamin E in a dropper bottle. Warm to body temperature and apply a half dropperful into the ear. Massage the ear canal for a minute or so. Let your pet shake its head and then gently clean out the canal with cotton swabs. Apply the oil every other day for six days. Then let the ears rest for three days. The oil mixture smothers mites and initiates a healing process.

Step 2: Dilute a tincture of the herb yellow dock by putting 9 drops in 1 tablespoon of water. Treat the ears with this mixture, as above, once every three days for six weeks. Ear mite eggs are quite resistant after they have hardened. For this reason it is necessary to undertake this step. The eggs will hatch out in cycles. If the medicine is present for six continuous weeks, the mites will be eliminated.

Step 3: Thoroughly shampoo the head and ears every two days for at least two to three times to eliminate any mites that may have ventured out from the ears. Also shampoo the tip of the tail, which may have acquired mites when curled near the head. Make a tea infusion of yellow dock, cool it down, and use it as a final rinse.

Ayurvedic Herb for Mites—Tejinder Sodhi, DVM

Neem oil is a powerful antifungal and antiparasitic herbal Ayurvedic agent derived from the neem tree (*Azaradichta indica*) in India. It is highly beneficial for cats and generally eliminates the problem without the need to use any toxic insecticide. It is available through Ayush Herbs (800-925-1371). If this doesn't help, see your veterinarian.

DOSAGE
- 5 to 10 drops twice daily in the affected ears for a week. Skip a week and repeat treatment. Skip another week and repeat.

⩗ Epilepsy (Seizures) ⩗

Epileptic seizures, also known as convulsions, are not as common in cats as in dogs. They are caused by an abnormal functioning in the brain—a kind of short circuit—where electrical impulses go haywire. This results in two types of seizures. One is called a "petit mal," characterized by spasm in a leg or one or more groups of muscles without a loss of consciousness. "Grand mal," the more severe type, causes loss of consciousness along with more generalized spasm. During an episode, which can last up to five minutes, there may be jerking, salivating, and loss of bladder control. A cat may appear confused and exhausted afterward.

Epilepsy is a complex issue, and there is usually not just one simple answer to it. Genetics, toxic exposures, allergies, and trauma may all play a role.

The conventional approach is to administer central nervous depressants—such as phenobarbital—for the remainder of a patient's life. Holistic veterinarians use combinations of acupuncture, diet, herbs, flower essences, and nutritional supplements to counteract epilepsy. Depending on the severity of the condition, they may be able to lessen or even eliminate the need for medication with these methods. Frequently it requires an integrated approach—using holistic measures and drugs—to control the seizures.

One area to pursue with your veterinarian is the allergy connection. Research has shown that seizures may be caused by food sensitivities (see section on food allergies). "Many times there are underlying food allergies involved with epilepsy," says Maria Glinski, DVM. "Avoid foods with preservatives, coloring, or chemical additives. Serve your animals top-quality food or homemade meals to help reduce the severity of this condition."

FLOWER ESSENCES
(See chapter 10 for general information on essences.)

Rescue Remedy for Seizures—Carolyn S. Blakey, DVM

Rescue Remedy, or Five Flower Remedy, as it is also called, is an effective and safe tool that pet owners can use to stop seizures. This well-known flower essence often works immediately. Keep the liquid remedy handy if you have an animal with a history of seizures. Give it when a seizure develops. Better yet, give it when you see the telltale signs of an episode. Such signs are variable: animals may become wobbly, clingy, or "spacey"; they may be wanting to hide, or they may suddenly develop the seizure.

With this remedy a seizure can often be aborted before it starts. Many of my clients tell me they are able to reduce the number of seizures by up to a half and minimize the intensity and duration of episodes. Animals are back to normal much quicker.

Rescue Remedy is not a cure. It buys time while you seek a more permanent solution with your veterinarian, whether it is controlling the problem with drugs or individualized holistic treatments such as acupuncture, herbs, and homeopathic medicines. There are generally no quick and easy answers. Seizures are a deep problem.

DOSAGE
- A few drops in an animal's mouth or lift the lip away from the teeth and squirt a few drops onto the gums.

HERBS

Valerian Root—Maria Glinski, DVM

If your animal still has seizures after you make dietary changes in an attempt to eliminate possible food allergies, I recommend the herb valerian root. Valerian is well-known for its activity on nervous disorders. In mild cases I can usually control seizures with valerian alone.

The product I use is the glycerin-based liquid drops made by Gaia Herbs (800-831-7780), available in health food stores. Cats are not tranquilized by valerian, but they may get a little sleepy if you give too much. So go slow if you increase the dose.

For more severe cases, or if the valerian is not enough, I will add acupuncture and individualized Chinese herbs. If I have to use phenobarbital, the natural approach is powerful enough so that only a minimum dose of the medication is needed.

DOSAGE
- Start with 5 drops twice a day and increase to 10 if needed. Do not increase the dose if the animal seems to be getting drowsy.

Chinese Herbs—Stan Gorlitsky, DVM

Many years ago I found a traditional Chinese multiherb formula that features bupleurum, a root with a long reputation for healing the liver. Working with an herbalist, I made a few modifications to the formula. The result is a formula I call Bupleurum 12 Combination, available through my clinic (803-881-9915). The product comes in powder form and is mixed into an animal's food.

The combination has a strong calming effect on the nervous system and can often on its own dramatically reduce the intensity and frequency of seizures. In addition, it protects the liver against toxicity and, in particular, against the buildup of drug toxicity from long-term use of phenobarbital for seizures. Animals frequently develop a tolerance to medication and require higher dosages for control. As a result they may become lethargic. With this formula I can usually reduce the amount of medication needed to control seizures. Sometimes I can eliminate medication totally.

If you want to try this formula, work with your veterinarian. Do not reduce medication on your own.

DOSAGE
- Follow label instructions.

NUTRITIONAL SUPPLEMENTS

Taurine for Early Cases—Karen Bentley, DVM

I use a variety of natural remedies for seizures depending on the individual condition. For an animal who has just started developing seizures and not been on too much medication, the amino acid taurine by itself can often abort epileptic episodes and help diminish the intensity of seizures. You can give it long-term.

Taurine, in many cases, seems to eliminate seizures altogether. This suggests to me that taurine deficiencies may be involved. So many animals have questionable beginnings and poor nutrition right from day one. Even though taurine has been supplemented in cat food, some animals probably have a need for even higher levels than what is contained in the food.

I recall the case of a kitten who was found in a ditch by the side of the road. The woman who found him brought the cat to my clinic. He was about four months old and had some back and spinal injury, suggesting he had been thrown from a car. I gave him some homeopathic remedies for the trauma. About three days later the cat started developing seizures. I then recommended taurine—a 500-milligram capsule three times daily. Gradually, over a two-month period, the seizures diminished in intensity and frequency and then stopped completely. We tried to cut back on the dosage, to 2 capsules a day, but the cat then started tremoring. The cat has now been maintained for four years on 1,500 milligrams of taurine daily. Some animals with a tendency for seizures may require that much for a lifetime.

DOSAGE
- 500-milligram capsule, two to three times daily.

Taurine Plus B-Complex Vitamins—Jean Hofve, DVM
I treat my cases with the amino acid taurine, along with a combination of two B-complex vitamins—B_6 and niacinamide (a form of niacin)—made by Standard Process (800-848-5061; sold through veterinarians). The combination tablet contains 50 milligrams of B_6 and 10 milligrams of niacinamide. I have very few repeat seizures after starting this simple regimen. The supplements are added to food.

DOSAGE
- **Taurine:** 125 milligrams daily.

- **B_6 and niacinamide combination:** 1 a day.

MIXED AND MISCELLANEOUS APPROACHES

Is Your Cat Overdosing on Light?—Lynne Friday, DVM

Be aware of the light source around animals with neurological problems, particularly epilepsy. Too much or too little light can exacerbate their problem.

An example of too much is constant exposure to the television screen. Animals are much better off without TV. Keep them away from Nintendo games as well. Intense rapid-eye images and furiously flickering screens generate too much stimulation for the brain and lower the ability of a cat's nervous system to counteract seizures, whatever the actual cause may be. In short, TV simply lowers your pet's neurological threshold. This is a serious consideration if you have a sensitive animal.

Install full-spectrum lighting where your animal spends much time. Cats with epilepsy may be light-sensitive. Their condition may become aggravated during the shorter days of winter. If your animal experiences more seizures between October and March, the problem may very well be due to shorter light days. You may be leaving lights on in the house, but the lights are generally of the incandescent and fluorescent type. Full-spectrum lights are more natural. They stimulate the body's production of melatonin, the hormone that governs the internal biological clock overseeing hormonal secretions, the sleep cycle, and repair and rejuvenation activities. Use the same full-spectrum lights you get for growing plants. Make sure the animal has access to them. You will find that animals will spend considerable time under the light if they have a light deficiency. You will also find they have fewer seizures.

⚓ Eye Problems ⚓

Regular physical examinations are a must for animals, and if any problem is developing in the eyes, the veterinarian should be able to pick it up. If you detect something going on in one or both eyes, point it out to your veterinarian.

"Don't take chances," says Carvel Tiekert, DVM. "Eyes can go blind very quickly. A severely red eye or an eye closed shut should be seen by a veterinarian. It may not appear to be serious, but don't take a chance. I have seen eyes lost because people waited twelve hours too long."

HERBS AND NUTRITIONAL SUPPLEMENTS

Nourish the Liver to Help the Eyes—Ron Carsten, DVM

Cleansing and nourishing the liver usually helps most chronic eye conditions that have not responded well to drug therapies. The basis for this approach stems from Chinese medicine, which describes a strong connection between the liver and the eyes.

I consistently see better results by adding a simple program with milk thistle, the herb that detoxifies the liver, and glutamine, an amino acid that nourishes the intestinal tract, which in turn eases the burden on the liver. Give supplements with meals.

Dosage
- **Milk thistle:** 250 milligrams twice a day.

- **Glutamine:** Glutamine, 500 milligrams twice a day for all animals.

Lysine for Herpes of the Eyes—Jean Hofve, DVM

Cats often develop a herpes virus condition in the eyeballs. It causes a conjunctivitis, an inflammation of the inside lining of the eyelids, and shallow, painful ulcers. The eyes will water and develop a copious, puslike discharge. The cat will squint.

The following remedies are useful:
1. The amino acid L-lysine. People take it to help control herpes outbreaks. You can use it for cats as well. I find that about half of the animals I recommend this for clear up to some degree, if not totally, on lysine.

    The problem may be related to stress. If you know your cat becomes stressed from certain situations, such as when you go away for a weekend, use the lysine preventively before you leave.
2. I also recommend artificial tears—but not the kind for contact lenses. The product should contain the ingredient methyl cellulose, sometimes called "hydroxy-methyl-cellulose." These drops

help wash away viral particles. The methyl cellulose enhances adherence of the drops on the eye, so you don't have to repeat the process that often. I have had success with a brand called Tears Renewed. These products are available in drugstores. They are also helpful as a preventive agent for cats with constantly weepy eyes, such as is frequently seen with Persians.

Caution: If the problem persists for more than a day or two, or if the discharge is thick, yellowish, or greenish, see a veterinarian. Ulcers can cause the loss of an eye. If the problem is chronic and has been diagnosed as herpes, use the lysine and eyedrops as a safe therapeutic measure. Some veterinarians may want to use antibiotics, but they will not help against this condition.

DOSAGE

- **Lysine:** 250 to 500 milligrams twice a day for up to five days for an acute episode. Break open the capsule and mix the contents into the food.

- **Artificial tears:** 1 or 2 drops, three or four times a day.

⌇ Feline Leukemia (FELV) ⌇

See Infectious Illnesses

⌇ Feline Infectious Peritonitis (FIP) ⌇

See Infectious Illnesses

≫ First Aid ≪

FLOWER ESSENCES
(See chapter 10 for general information on essences.)

Rescue Remedy to the Rescue—Carolyn Blakey, DVM

For any kind of trauma, stress, or shock, whether emotional, mental, or physical, I recommend Rescue Remedy, also known as Five Flower Remedy. This well-known flower essence remedy is available at health food stores. Keep it handy at home, in your purse, in your car, in your office. It is an amazing natural medicine for calming both people and animals.

Once a cat owner brought in his comatose animal who had gotten into a yellow jacket nest and been stung repeatedly. I removed the remaining yellow jackets and over the next several hours gave the remedy four or five times to the cat directly in its mouth. That's all I did in this case. The cat recovered quickly.

DOSAGE
- A few drops in the mouth or rubbed onto the head of the animal. In critical situations, the remedy can be given repeatedly.

WEEDS FOR WOUNDS

Plantain, also known as "ribwort" or "white man's foot," is a common weed that offers healing and antiseptic benefits when applied to superficial wounds, infections, stings, bites, or localized itchiness (such as poison oak or ivy) or when used to help draw toxins or splinters to the surface of the skin. Boil plantain leaves in water. Dip a washcloth and apply as a warm poultice over the affected site. A perfect time to use it would be if you notice a puncture wound or scratch right after a cat fight. Use it several times a day for a few minutes each time if possible or as often as you can while there is a problem. If the wound worsens, be sure to see a veterinarian.

HOMEOPATHIC REMEDIES
(See chapter 9 for general information on homeopathics.)

Arnica for Trauma—Charles Loops, DVM

The amazing results consistently experienced with the use of Arnica after trauma gets more people interested in homeopathy than any other remedy. Arnica is a magnificent remedy for pain, shock, bruising, contusion, animal fights, or bites. It should be the first remedy you reach for. It will stop bleeding, arrest shock, reduce pain, and remove anxiety associated with injury and surgery (see section on surgery). The sooner it can be given after injury, the better the response. Keep a supply in your first-aid kit, car, workshop, kitchen, and bathroom.

Arnica 30C will work for just about every situation. For life-threatening, major shock situations, higher potencies of 200C or 1M have amazing results. I have seen Arnica at such high potencies literally keep animals alive who were severely injured by automobiles. If they do succumb to their injuries, they do so much more peacefully.

DOSAGE
- Repeat doses as needed. Immediately after trauma, a dose can be given every few minutes. The farther removed from the trauma, the less frequently the remedy is given.

Arnica Gel—Robert Goldstein, VMD

If you want double the healing help, use Arnica gel topically along with the homeopathic remedy orally. Arnica gel contains *Arnica montana*, a plant with a great healing history against bruises, aches, and pains. The brand I use is ArniFlora, made by Boricke and Tafel, available at health food stores and even some pharmacies.

Apply the gel up to four times daily (externally only) for bumps, bruises, swelling, or joints that are stiff from overexertion or arthritis. Part the hair and gently rub the gel directly on the skin. Avoid getting it into the eyes, and do not use the product if there is any break in the skin. If pain or swelling appears to worsen or persist for more than two or three days, see your veterinarian.

Calendula for Cuts and Raw Skin—A. Greig Howie, DVM

Calendula (marigold) is a remarkable healing agent. I am amazed at how fast it works for scratches, cuts, and raw skin. Calendula ointments, or liquid mother tinctures, are readily available in health food stores. If you use the liquid form, put a dropperful in a cup of water with a pinch of salt to clean out a wound. Don't use it for puncture wounds, because it may heal the top of the wound too fast and leave the infection below. There is no problem if an animal licks it off after you apply it.

MIXED AND MISCELLANEOUS APPROACHES

Stop Bleeding with Pepper—Stan Gorlitsky, DVM

If an animal incurs a minor bleeding wound or cut, sprinkle on some common cayenne pepper from your kitchen spice rack. Pepper enhances the clotting process and helps to stop the bleeding.

Comfrey for Fractures—Norman C. Ralston, DVM

Use comfrey to help speed bone healing. It is available in different forms: homeopathic remedies, herbal tinctures, and powders and capsules. Comfrey can be used internally or as a poultice applied directly to an affected area. It can make a dramatic difference for slow-healing breaks.

⫸ Fleas and Insect Bites ⫷

The flea, and specifically a protein in the flea saliva, is the number one source of allergic reactions in cats. For a sensitive cat, even a single bite from a single flea can cause turmoil internally in the immune system and externally on the skin. Flea allergy dermatitis is the typical result—a cat itchy all over and scratching incessantly. Sometimes a cat will chew and scratch on one spot and create bald patches of irritated skin.

Holistic veterinarians often comment that healthy animals are

less likely to be "flea magnets." The key to resistance, they emphasize, is feeding a superior diet (see chapters 3 to 6 in part 1).

As William Pollak, DVM, says: "The best flea control is a vital
animal that radiates health and fitness, an animal consuming fresh,
wholesome food and living in a good, natural balance with its environment. The presence of fleas is an indication that you need to create greater life energy in your pet."

Joseph Demers, DVM, practices in Florida, where conditions of
heat, dampness, and sandy soil make the state a paradise for fleas.
Nevertheless, he says, "I have found that cats who are healthy just
don't attract the fleas, or if they do, it is minimal. The same holds
true with the wild animals who are brought in. The weak ones are
full of fleas, ticks, and parasites. The stronger ones are much less
affected. The way to develop a strong, healthy animal is first and
foremost good nutrition."

FLEAS

Natural vs. Advantage—Robert Goldstein, VMD

I have spoken to both holistic and conventional veterinarians about
Advantage and similar products. The consensus is that these are relatively safe and a vast improvement over the older generation of
products derived from nerve gas (organic phosphate poisons) that
had overt, proven negative health effects.

My advice is to use natural approaches first, and if they work, fine.
But if you have a continuing problem, use Advantage, which appears
to be the best of these products according to my research. However,
it is not for every animal. If your animal is older, debilitated, or bat-
tling an acute or chronic disease, such as cancer, don't use it.

With any chemically based product, there may be some side
effects in a small number of cases. A local, transient rash or irritation is the most common. Rarely, an animal might go off feed,
vomit, or show increased thirst, urination, or diarrhea. If these signs
occur, stop using the product and consult your veterinarian at once.

First, though, give natural methods a fair chance. I recommend
Internal Powder, available through Earth Animal at 800-711-2292.
This product is a formula I developed nearly twenty years ago that
contains unprocessed brewer's yeast and mineral-rich ingredients.

Follow the label instructions. It can be mixed with yogurt and then blended into your dog's food. You can safely double the dose on the label to gear up for flea season.

Garlic is another useful flea deterrent, as well as an all-around immune system and cardiovascular "tonic." If you don't like the odor it produces, add some chopped parsley.

To boost the natural program from the outside, I am a longtime fan of a product called 100% Natural Flea and Tick Repellent, made by Quantum Herbal Products and available through the manufacturer (800-348-0398) or Earth Animal.

I also recommend Cloud Nine Herbal Dip by Halo (800-426-4256). It is safe and easy to use and contains powerful aromatic herbs (pine needle, peppermint, tea tree oil, rosemary, sage, and eucalyptus) that will last a good month on your animal's body. It can be used as a dip or spray or added for antiflea power to your favorite shampoo.

If your animal is still plagued by fleas after using these kinds of natural approaches, I suggest turning to Advantage. Use it only as often as necessary. Many of my clients stretch the dose to every six weeks and find no falloff in effectiveness.

When to Use the New Flea Products—Carvel Tiekert, DVM

Over the years, I haven't found that natural products work well in the face of a severe flea problem. I have a huge number of satisfied clients using Advantage, Program, or Frontline, the new pharmaceutical antiflea medications. Many of these pet owners previously tried natural products and suffered through the constant warfare. The new products appear safe and effective. I have encountered only one animal who had a skin reaction.

I don't push the pharmaceutical products because I don't think they are necessary in most cases. I suggest waiting until there is a problem before starting them. If a problem develops, first try brewer's yeast, which works for some animals, or garlic, or some other natural flea control product available at pet and health food stores.

Frontline and Advantage kill the fleas on the animal. Program sterilizes the fleas. If you have an animal sensitive to flea bites, Program won't provide immediate relief because the fleas are still aboard. Eventually it will help, since you won't have hatching eggs to renew the cycle, and the number of symptom-producing flea bites will be significantly reduced. However, if the animal ranges over any territory of consequence where it can attract a new crop of fleas, then Program is virtually useless.

As for collars, herbal or otherwise, they aren't effective in my experience.

Don't forget regular combing of the hair coat. The flea comb is the most important thing an owner can use to determine whether the flea battle is being won or lost.

Natural Remedies for Fleas—Joseph Demers, DVM

A combination of brewer's yeast and garlic may be helpful, as long as the animal isn't sensitive to the yeast. If scratching intensifies after you start brewer's yeast, then you know it's not the right thing for your pet.

You can help control fleas inside your house by using boric acid products on your carpets and floors, and outside with nematodes and diatomaceous earth. These products are widely available in health food and pet stores. Follow label instructions.

Make it your routine to regularly bathe, brush, and comb your animal. If your animal is healthy, these simple measures can go a long way to minimize the presence of fleas.

For flea and other insect bites, the homeopathic remedies Apis mellifica and Rhus tox often provide relief within twenty-four hours from the usual scratching.

> DOSAGE
> - **Apis mellifica 6C:** Give up to five times daily if there is a raised red bump at the site of the bite.
>
> - **Rhus tox 6C:** Give up to five times daily if there is less sign of inflammation.

Fleas Flee from Flowers—Carolyn Blakey, DVM

For situations where your animal is bothered by a few fleas and there is no major infestation, and you don't want to use a poison, try Flee Free, a liquid flower essence remedy from Molly Sheehan's

Green Hope Farms (603-469-3662). You can use it as a spray or give directly to the animal.

DOSAGE
- Follow label instructions.

Nontoxic Dip—Lynne Friday, DVM

If you need to resort to a dip, I have found an excellent nontoxic product that works well for virtually all patients, whether they are very young or very old. It is called LymDyp S and is a ready-to-use solution of sulfurated lime that leaves a nice scent on the animal. It is available through DVM Pharmaceuticals, Inc. (305-575-6200), but needs to be ordered for you by your veterinarian.

DOSAGE
- Follow label instructions.

TICKS AND OTHER INSECT BITES

Homeopathic Ledum—Michelle Yasson, DVM

The homeopathic remedy Ledum is excellent for any kind of puncture wound in general, including cat bite wounds or tick bites. If your animal gets a tick, remove the insect and use the Ledum.

Echinacea is also useful as a natural immune booster, and I recommend it for cases of tick bite. I prefer the capsule form, which is tasteless and can be mixed right into the food.

DOSAGE
- **Ledum 30C:** Once within twenty-four hours of removing the tick. If the tick is engorged with blood, this is an indication that the insect has been present longer. In such cases, give Ledum once a day for two days.

- **Echinacea:** One-quarter of the human dose for five days.

FOR OTHER INSECTS

For insect bites and sudden swelling, I suggest the homeopathic remedy Apis mellifca. Apis is good for situations involving swelling. Many times you see the swelling go down after the first dose.

DOSAGE
- **Apis 30C:** Once may be enough, but can be repeated as often as every ten minutes for a total of four doses if needed.

Ledum for Spider Bites—Charles Loops, DVM

Spider bites usually produce a local hard swelling without heat. If you suspect a bite of this nature, Ledum is a good remedy.

DOSAGE
- **Ledum 30C:** Twice daily for two or three days or until the swelling disappears.

⌁ Food Allergies ⌁

See also Digestive Disorders

A healthy animal may not have trouble eating most foods. However, if you feed the same food daily for years, there is potential for intolerances to develop—particularly if the diet consists of a cheap commercial pet food containing multiple ingredients of poor quality.

Typical reactions involve vomiting, diarrhea, and scratching. Food allergies may also manifest as poor absorption of nutrients. Each animal is individual. There are many potential reactions. Two hypersensitive cats may react differently to the same food depending on their individual weaknesses and strengths.

Any animal can become allergic to any food—a protein source, a fruit, a vegetable. Just a small amount of an offending food could be enough to trigger reactions in some animals. In others, reactions occur from constantly feeding the same food.

Experts say that food allergies are less a problem among cats than dogs. The incidence is estimated at between 5 and 15 percent of cats.

Foods "High in Trouble"—"The HIT List"—Alfred Plechner, DVM

(Note: Food allergy expert Alfred Plechner, DVM, was a co-creator of the first lamb and rice diet, marketed by Nature's Recipe, and also helped design the company's line of special diets for food-sensitive animals.)

Based on years of treating animals for food allergy-related disorders, I created an allergic HIT list of major food offenders. These are the foods that set off the alarm most frequently—that is, cause the most trouble in sensitive animals. You may have a cat that is sensitive to any one or several of them.

The HIT list below may shock you. You may be thinking, "There is nothing left to feed my sensitive animal." Let me console you—there are plenty of foods you can prepare.

THE "HIT LIST"

1. Beef and beef by-products.
2. Milk. In my experience, perhaps up to 80 percent of animals, no matter what age, cannot tolerate cow's milk. After drinking it, they usually have gassy stomachs, vomiting, loose stool, or diarrhea. Raw, low-fat, or nonfat—it doesn't matter. However, there is a much greater tolerance to cottage cheese, other cheeses, and yogurt.
3. Yeast, yeast-containing foods, brewer's yeast (as given to animals for supposed flea protection. Unfortunately, I do see quite a few animals sensitive to yeast).
4. Corn and corn oil.
5. Pork.
6. Turkey.
7. Eggs. Yes, they can be allergenic, particularly the whites. Years ago, egg embryos were used in preparing distemper vaccines for dogs, but they were dropped from the formulations when it was found that they caused allergic reactions in many animals.
8. Fish and fish oils. If you want to provide omega-3 fatty acids to your animal, use plant oils instead, such as flaxseed oil.
9. Wheat and wheat by-products (when in combination with other allergens).
10. Soybeans. This used to be a fine source of protein, but now many animals can't handle it. Tofu, the fermented soybean product, is less allergenic, but nevertheless some animals are sensitive to it.
11. Chicken.

In order to help affected animals who seemingly have fewer food options open to them, I worked with Nature's Recipe eight years ago to develop what are called "limited antigen diets." The idea was to combine potatoes with protein sources that animals had little exposure to and that were thus less likely to cause problems.

Testing validated the concept, leading to the production of a number of dry and canned foods for dogs and cats called Innovative Veterinary Diets. Each item has just two ingredients—one source of protein and one source of carbohydrate—so as to limit the potential for allergic reaction. Such foods include lamb, duck, rabbit, or venison along with potatoes. We have found that animals tend to be less allergic to white potatoes than even rice.

The recommendation is to use a particular food for four to six months and then switch to another. For example, you feed duck and potatoes for four months, then switch to rabbit and potatoes. These foods are widely available on a prescription basis from veterinarians for animals with food disorders. For additional vitamins, minerals, and enzymes, I recommend adding fresh vegetables and fruits to the base food and a good nutritional supplement. The supplement I recommend is Power for Life, made by Terra Oceana (805-563-2634). It contains a health-boosting range of vitamins, trace minerals, enzymes, and whole-food factors. Follow label instructions.

When a cat develops signs of intolerance to foods, the problem may be linked to an endocrine-immune dysfunction, a genetic fallout from years of inbreeding and line breeding. Among other things, this can create an erratic metabolism and intolerance to many foods. When certain hormones go awry, they fail to properly regulate the immune system. In the digestive tract, uncontrolled immune cells challenge food components as foreign invaders, setting off a whole scenario of upset, intolerance, and malabsorption, resulting in animals not being able to extract adequate nutrition from the food.

As genetic defects become perpetuated in the gene pool of breeding stock, it appears that more and more animals are able to tolerate fewer and fewer foods. With some severely affected animals, unless you correct their deep-seated hormone-antibody levels with replacement therapy, there is hardly anything left they can eat. This may sound overly dramatic, but the reality in my practice is that I see more pets in this sad shape now than before—and I have been studying this problem for many years. The situation has become worse, and many animals are dying early in life because of it. In my opinion we have entered into a genetic ice age (in chapter 15, Plechner describes a blood test that can determine such imbalances and what can be done to correct them).

TIPS FOR FEEDING SAFER FOODS

If you have a food-intolerant animal, the following suggestions can help minimize problems:

- Always read the ingredient label. The shorter the list, the better. The longer the list, the greater the chance of encountering an offending ingredient. Keep in mind that the first three ingredients on the label usually make up 90 percent of the contents.

- Try to avoid the ingredients on the HIT list, foods that often cause reactions in susceptible animals.

- Look out for, and avoid, products with chemical additives. This means the artificial colors, artificial flavors, artificial sweeteners, preservatives, and stabilizers. All have the potential to intensify or wholly activate an allergic reaction.

- Fresh and wholesome foods are, of course, much better for your animal, as they are for us. But they, too, have the potential to cause reactions because of hormonal-immune imbalances. This includes raw meat. The food may be great, but your animal just may not be able to tolerate it.

THE ADD-BACK PLAN

If you know or feel that your cat has an intolerance problem, but you don't know what the particular offending food or foods are, try the following strategy:

- For one week, feed lamb meat or a baby food containing pure lamb meat. Cats tolerate lamb quite well. For this test or long-term for a sensitive animal, you can use any of the Innovative Veterinary Diet products available through veterinarians.

- If the stools are good, and there are no signs of food intolerance such as itching, scratching, stomach upset, or diarrhea, do a slow add-back of foods, one at a time, and each for a week before you add a new food. You might want to try home-prepared chicken the second week, then a white fish or tuna (for human consumption) in spring water.

- Again, if there are no problems, you can begin to test commercial canned pet foods. Test one a week. Give each food you try a seven-day trial. As foods pass the test, you will begin to build up a "safe list" of items that can be fed.

- Continue to add back any food to the regular diet after it has passed the test. You can then rotate, mix, and ad-lib within the boundaries of tolerated food. In this way, you will soon develop an individualized hypoallergenic menu for your animal.

- Include raw vegetables such as carrots and celery, if your cat will eat them.

- If you choose to add a commercial kibble, be alert for reactions. Remember that many commercial foods have multiple ingredients of poor quality, along with chemical additives, that increase the potential for trouble. Select a quality product, such as one of the better "natural" brands available in health food stores or pet nutrition centers. Look for a product with as short a list of ingredients as possible.

- Eliminate any nutritional supplements and snacks when you are testing. In this plan, all foods and even ingredients in nutritional supplements are guilty until proven innocent. Later, once you have a firm handle on a problem-free diet, you can slowly begin to reintroduce supplements. But monitor them as you would the food.

- For variety, it's okay to share what you eat with your cat—if your cat will eat it. Any kind of meat, unseasoned pastas, vegetables, and salad can be added to the base diet. But if your animal starts to scratch, vomits or has diarrhea, or becomes lethargic, then the light bulb should go on. You may have fed something that your animal cannot tolerate. So be watchful and use common sense if you have a sensitive animal.

Limit the Number of Foods You Feed—Nancy Scanlan, DVM

I prefer to try to limit the number of meats and grains present in the diet so you can more easily fall back on a different food source if a food allergy does develop. You may have to go to a mono diet, where you start with one food and then add others slowly to test for sensitivity.

Some people make the error of feeding a special hypoallergenic diet and then continue giving a treat that has ingredients an animal may be allergic to, such as dairy or beef. Watch out for the "extras" you give your animals, including table scraps. They can cause problems just as much as the daily entrée.

Food Allergy or Quality Allergy?—William Pollak, DVM

Diets that contain poor and inappropriate ingredients—unfortunately this represents a good deal of what is sold as commercial pet food—create animals who do not function properly. Their systems are continually besieged with toxicity. Under this constant burden, even otherwise harmless and beneficial nutrients become part of a cascade of events that unleashes an internal "attack" mode against the food. The symptoms that arise from this we say are related to food allergies. We blame the individual ingredients.

Allergy in all its forms is a reflection of a system starving for higher nutrition and health. An appropriate diet for an individual animal is soothing, nourishing, and a source of wellness, orderliness, intelligence, and vital life energy for the body. A diet of fresh, varied, and wholesome food, along with vitamin and mineral supplementation, offers the nutrients that create health and vitality and eliminates allergy and disease. Rather than eliminating food and dealing with food allergies on the level of illness, feed a better diet and operate from the level of wellness. This approach works for a large majority of animals.

Poor Meat Quality Equals Allergies—Jean Hofve, DVM

Food allergies among humans tend to involve things like dairy, wheat, and citrus, and virtually no one seems sensitive to meat. Yet much of the problem with pets appears to be related to meat. No wonder, because meat used in pet foods is a far cry from the meat an animal would eat in a natural state. Pet food meat sources may be cancerous or spoiled to begin with and then goes through processing that denatures the enzymes and adulterates the proteins. If you feed a commercial food diet, look for brands that have no chemical additives listed on the label. Find a food that your animal tolerates and then slowly add as much good additional food as you can, such as raw meat and vegetables.

⚓ Gum Disease ⚓

See Dental Health

⚓ Hairballs ⚓

Cats are uniquely fastidious and spend a good deal of time pursuing the instinctual feline act of self-grooming. The digestive tract normally takes care of small amounts of hair that are swallowed and passes them out with the stool. Now and then a cat may naturally vomit up a hairball. However, if an overload of fur is ingested, the cat may not be able to eliminate the hair from either end. If they become large enough, hairballs can cause constipation and bowel obstruction and, in severe cases, require surgical removal.

You tend to see more problems with long-haired cats and animals who have parasites or skin allergies. Severely allergic cats, in fact, may sometimes lick off most of their fur, leaving hair only on their head, a strip along their spine, and a bit on the tail. More frequently, such cats may lick bare the surface of their undersides and parts of their chests.

Holistic veterinarians say that these problems are infrequent when cats eat a good diet. You will also see fewer hairball problems if you take a minute or two every day to brush your cat. Brushing removes loose and dead hairs before they are swallowed and thus minimizes the potential for hairballs. In addition, brushing puts you in regular intimate contact with your adopted companion. This is another good way to become more familiar with your cat and monitor subtle health changes.

Excessive hair shedding, and a higher risk of hairballs, may be experienced by indoor cats exposed to continual dry, hot-air heating.

Herbal Relief from Constipation—Paul McCutcheon, DVM

Does your cat have constipation from hairballs? If that is the case, try a natural supplement called Herbolax, made by Seroyal Inc. (800-263-5861; sold through health professionals). The supplement quickly clears up the constipation. Whatever you do, however, make an effort to find the cause of the problem. If your cat's skin is dry, the animal may benefit from an essential fatty acid supplement.

DOSAGE

• **Herbolax:** 1/2 to 1 tablet daily, depending on the size of the cat.

Shedding and Intestinal Relief—Stan Gorlitsky, DVM

Lax-eze is a powder formula with sea minerals, bentonite clay, dried beet pulp, psyllium seed husks, and enzymes that goes to work quickly after it is eaten by an animal. It is available through Good Communications (800-968-1738).

The product maximizes digestion and absorption of food, cleans the intestinal tract, produces a lustrous coat, and dramatically reduces shedding. Hairball problems in cats have been reported to disappear rapidly.

I developed Lax-eze more than fifteen years ago and have used it successfully for many hundreds of animals in my own practice. Other veterinarians have used it with equal success. The formula is also helpful to stop constipation and diarrhea.

DOSAGE

• Sprinkle on food. It has a liver flavor that pets enjoy. Follow label instructions.

Psyllium Plus Digestive Enzymes—Nancy Scanlan, DVM

To help cats pass the hairballs, use a pinch of psyllium powder, available at health food stores, in combination with digestive enzymes.

Mix into the food. Do this once or twice a day during shedding season or whenever you see hair coming through. This combination helps push the hair through the system, but you need to fix the problem causing hairballs in the first place. Long-haired cats should be brushed daily. Allergies and parasites should be treated appropriately.

Butter Relief—Alfred Plechner, DVM

A simple remedy to try at the outset of a hairball problem is to put a tad of butter on the roof of the cat's mouth or somewhere on the body where the animal will lick it off. You can also add a very small bit of flax oil in the food. The idea is to provide extra lubrication to carry the hair through and out the other end.

Metamucil—Lynne Friday, DVM

I once treated a cat who ate an ornament off the Christmas tree. I told the owner to feed it Metamucil. The pieces went right through the cat like a tube of gelatin. The product works for hairballs as well.

Relief with Vaseline—Jean Hofve, DMV

Most hairball remedies are basically flavored Vaseline. They seem to work fine. I used simple Vaseline for my cat throughout her whole life, and she lived to be over twenty. It didn't hurt her a bit. For this purpose, Vaseline appears to be a benign substance that glues hair together and helps slide the hair out in the feces. It doesn't seem to be absorbed in the body. You can smush a bit into your cat's mouth or smear it thinly onto the fur of the shoulder or front leg, in an area that is easily accessible to the tongue. It will annoy the cat and be rapidly cleaned up. Don't put it on some unreachable part of the body where the cat will just rub it off on your furniture. Also don't just put a glob on their paw. They may shake it off and you'll find the glob stuck to your ceiling or television screen. Wait at least an hour after feeding before you apply the Vaseline so as not to interfere with the absorption of food in any way.

⚜ Heart Problems ⚜

If your cat shows any of the following signs, don't waste time in seeing your veterinarian; your cat may have advanced heart disease:

- Coughing, usually at night or upon arising.
- Wheezing, shortness of breath, panting at the least exertion.
- Potbelly or swollen limbs.
- Lack of energy and appetite, with continual sleeping and depression.
- Fainting, stumbling, or weakness, dragging of hind legs.
- Bluish gray lips, tongue, or gums.

These are signs of cardiomyopathy, a degeneration and failure of the heart muscle and the most common cardiac condition among cats.

Just as heart disease is a major killer among humans, it can be deadly to cats as well. And just like humans, cats benefit from regular checkups, too. An annual checkup is good insurance against heart disease. If the heart is ailing, early detection and prompt correction improve the prognosis.

Heart disease is not necessarily an "old cat" phenomenon. Many cats are growing old before their time with weakening hearts and impaired circulation. Veterinarians say, in fact, that heart problems have become increasingly prevalent at younger ages and commonly occur in middle-aged cats six to eight years old.

"Unlike the situation with humans, the problem is not a result of clogged arteries," says Robert Goldstein, VMD. "Heart disease among pets has other causes, such as an infectious agent (bacterial or viral), a run-down or stressed immune system, a genetic defect, and poor-quality nutrition. Unnecessary vaccines and exposure to environmental and chemical pollutants also contribute."

For an existing heart condition, follow your veterinarian's therapeutic program, which generally includes a variety of medications. Alternative and conventional therapies used in concert can be quite effective. If a cat has advanced disease, the drugs may keep the animal alive long enough for good diet, nutritional supplements, and other natural remedies to kick in and have a restorative, strengthening effect on the body. Depending on the severity of the condition, the natural approach may allow for the reduction, or even elimination, of medications. Ideally, consult with a holistic veterinarian to structure an effective cardiac program using natural methods. Such veterinarians often recommend acupuncture for animals with heart problems. The technique helps rebalance the body and remove energy blockages.

From a nutritional standpoint, the amino acid taurine has for years been linked to a condition called "dilated cardiomyopathy." In dilated cardiomyopathy, the heart muscle tissue thins out and enlarges. This causes the heart valves to leak and leads to heart failure. Cats are very sensitive to a deficiency of taurine, which is found in meat and fish. If it is deficient in the diet, it can be an underlying cause of cardiomyopathy. Many commercial cat foods, particularly cheaper ones, may be deficient owing to poor-quality protein sources, such as tendons, cartilage, and other beef or chicken byproducts. Premium cat foods that use whole meat and chicken are most likely to have adequate levels.

"The minimum amount of taurine in commercial pet food has been raised twice in recent years because of heart problems in cats," says Nancy Scanlan, DVM. "Yet we still see problems from eating this food. Taurine appears to remain an unresolved problem in cat nutrition. I believe supplementation is smart prevention against cardiomyopathy."

As you will read here, holistic veterinarians have a short list of cardiac-supporting supplement favorites. The main ones, besides taurine, are the following:

- **Coenzyme Q$_{10}$.** This fat-soluble vitamin, known as CoQ$_{10}$ for short, is widely recognized around the world as a major nutritional aid for ailing hearts. It contributes directly to the production of energy in all cells of the body. It gives a big boost to the around-the-clock energy requirements of the heart muscle. CoQ$_{10}$ is most effective when given with food that contains some fat.

- **Vitamin E.** This well-known vitamin improves circulation and cardiac output. Like CoQ_{10}, it is also an important antioxidant providing protection against molecular damage throughout the body caused by oxidation of cellular components.

- **L-carnitine.** This amino acid strengthens the heart muscle. It promotes weight loss in obese cats by helping the body to burn fat.

In this section you will see a variety of dosage recommendations. If you have any doubts about what is appropriate for your animal, always start low and increase the amount if necessary.

DO HEART PROBLEMS START IN THE MOUTH?— JAN BELLOWS, DVM

If your animal's teeth are not cleaned properly, you may face the risk of not just gum disease, but heart disease as well. Animals with bad gums are more prone to heart problems.

Bacterial infections originating in the gums can spread into the body and attack the heart valves. The result is a condition known as "bacterial endocarditis." It can be deadly. The disturbance to the tissue interferes with the proper function of the valves. Fluid may back up into the lungs and cause congestive heart failure.

Refer to the section on dental problems for information on how to keep your pet's mouth healthy.

NUTRITIONAL SUPPLEMENTS

Taurine—Karen Bentley, DVM

I find that taurine is always helpful, and for that reason I use a high, yet safe, level for my cardiac cats. I remember a two-year-old domestic shorthair named Bimbo who was kept alive for another seven years with diuretic therapy along with taurine.

Because there may be a genetic component to cardiomyopathy, taurine can also be used as a preventive supplement for siblings of affected cats.

DOSAGE
- 500 milligrams three times daily. Open capsule, mix into food.

Taurine, Vitamin E, and CoQ$_{10}$—Nancy Scanlan, DVM

Taurine, vitamin E, and coenzyme Q$_{10}$ alone may improve an animal's condition in some cases, but in others medication may be required. If they work alone, you should see improvement in a few days to a week—more energy and less blueness of the tongue, lips, or gums.

DOSAGE
- **Taurine:** If the animal is eating a commercial diet, 200 milligrams daily of taurine. If eating a home-prepared diet, then increase to 500 milligrams.

- **Vitamin E:** 50 IU daily.

- **CoQ$_{10}$:** 10 milligrams.

CoQ$_{10}$, Vitamin E, Carnitine, and Kelp—Robert Goldstein, VMD

Above all, feed the best possible diet. Then add to the food a number of excellent heart-specific nutrients—all readily available in health food stores. These nutrients can enhance your animal's prognosis and improve quality of life.

My heart supplement program includes CoQ$_{10}$, which, when given long-term, can lessen your animal's dependence on medication. It also encourages more exercise, improves circulation, and promotes weight loss in obese animals. The program also includes vitamin E, L-carnitine, and powdered kelp, an excellent source of minerals that supply the body's electrical system, which in turn keeps the heart pumping. Commercial pet foods are often deficient in minerals or contain minerals in a form that are poorly absorbed. Look for a deep, cold-water source of kelp at health food stores.

In case of the existence of a taurine deficiency in the diet, add this critical amino acid to the program.

Just like humans, cats need regular exercise, also. It improves general circulation. Ultimately the best answer for heart disease lies in prevention, where diet and exercise share the spotlight.

To create an individually tailored nutritional and remedy program for patients with heart disease and other serious, life-threatening conditions, I use a special test I developed years ago. The test is called the Bio-Nutritional Analysis and is available to veterinarians at 800-670-0830 (for more details see chapter 16).

DOSAGE

- **CoQ$_{10}$:** 10 to 30 milligrams daily.

- **Vitamin E:** 200 IU daily.

- **L-carnitine:** 250 milligrams daily.

- **Kelp:** 1/2 teaspoon per meal, mixed into food.

- **Taurine:** Small cats, up to five pounds, 250 milligrams; five pounds and above, 500 milligrams.

Vitamin E, Selenium, and CoQ$_{10}$—Roger DeHaan, DVM

After graduating from veterinary school thirty years ago, I started practicing under an older veterinarian who had followed the work of Wilfrid Shute, M.D., the Canadian pioneer of vitamin E for heart conditions. We used the vitamin along with selenium, a mineral also important for the heart. The results were quite dramatic. A cat or a dog would come in with a weakened heart, an enlarged heart, or a murmur, and we would start them on the supplements. A month later, when we saw them again, they were new animals, with more energy and clearly acting as if they were feeling better. I was never taught this in medical school, but I became a believer way back then and have been using this combination ever since for old animals and animals with weak hearts, cardiomyopathy, or any cardiac condition. More recently I added CoQ$_{10}$, the vitamin that perks up the heart muscle.

I suggest the following program if you want to try a holistic approach for heart problems, perhaps when the condition is not advanced enough to necessitate drugs or when drugs are causing problems. You can also use this to support any conventional treatment. Along with a good diet, you should see solid improvement within a month.

DOSAGE

- **Vitamin E** (preferably in the form of d-alpha tocopherol— natural vitamin E): 30 IU daily.

- **Selenium** (preferably in the form of selenium methionate): 30 micrograms daily.

- **CoQ$_{10}$:** 1 milligram per pound of body weight. Cut back to half dose for maintenance when animal improves.

Hawthorn and CoQ$_{10}$—A. Greig Howie, DVM

I recommend adding beef or lamb heart to the food of animals with heart conditions. Studies have shown that proteins from a particular organ meat will actually be utilized by that organ.

The primary supplement in my heart program is hawthorn, the herb that comes from Europe, where it is routinely prescribed by medical doctors and cardiologists to improve heart function. It is available here in health food stores. Be sure to purchase a product that contains a standardized extract of the herb.

Hawthorn is packed with potent compounds called vitexin, quercetin, and oligomeric procyanidins. These are phytochemicals—natural plant chemicals—that enhance the flow of blood to the heart and extremities and also promote the pumping action of the heart muscle.

I also use a good deal of CoQ$_{10}$, particularly for cardiomyopathy. I don't stop any prescriptive medication; however, over a few month's time an animal may improve enough on the combination so that medication can be reduced and perhaps even discontinued. But always work with a veterinarian, and do not stop medication on your own.

DOSAGE
- **Hawthorn:** Purchase a glycerine-based tincture. Add 4 to 6 drops three times a day. Put it in the food.

- **CoQ$_{10}$:** 5 to 10 milligrams daily.

⅏ Infectious Illnesses ⅏ (Viral and Upper-Respiratory Conditions)

Domestic cats are vulnerable to infectious illnesses that range from the common feline cold, characterized by sneezing bouts, to deadly viral conditions that can trigger cancer and a progressive AIDS-like loss of immunity. Stress, poor diet, and environmental toxins are major factors that undermine a cat's resistance. Genetics, of course, plays a big role. Some cats are simply more robust than others.

Holistic veterinarians emphasize good nutrition above all, with additional support from a supplement program, as the best way to keep animals healthy and resistant to the many germs that come their way. Supplement recommendations vary among practitioners but typically include a quality pet multi-vitamin/mineral formula with extra vitamins C and E and other antioxidants.

"The name of the game is prevention," says Wendell Belfield, DVM. "Cats on super nutrition have fewer infectious illnesses, and when they do come down with something it tends not to be as severe."

Cats, and particularly young ones, are susceptible to upper-respiratory infections that affect the nose, throat, and eyes, causing sneezing, coughing, fever, and runny eyes and noses. The condition can be as uncomplicated as a common cold with a few days of mild sneezing. It can, however, take on life-threatening proportions owing to secondary bacterial infections or if a cat loses its appetite and becomes malnourished and dehydrated. Sick cats will often fast for a couple of days. Be alert. Call your veterinarian for advice. Of the half dozen or so viruses that can cause upper-respiratory infections, the rhinotracheitis virus (also known as "the feline herpes virus") and the calicivirus have the most potential for harm. Many cats who carry these viruses may have recurrences of sneezing throughout their lives.

Cats are also threatened by a number of serious viruses that operate on a more systemic level:

- **Feline leukemia virus (FeLV).** This virus can cause anemia, diarrhea, or constipation, enlarged lymph nodes, loss of energy and appetite, infertility, and general suppression of immunity. Some infected cats also develop malignant masses and a dangerous lymph-related cancer called "lymphosarcoma." FeLV is regarded as the leading infectious killer disease among domestic cats; however, a large majority of cats exposed to the virus are able to muster enough immunity so that they do not become symptomatic. Such cats may be positive for the virus in lab tests but don't become sick and often live out their lives normally. The virus spreads from cat to cat primarily through saliva after prolonged and intensive contact between animals. Stress or immune-suppressing medication could open the door to the active disease process at some point. Symptomatic cats may live only weeks or months, depending on the individual strength of the animal.

- **Feline infectious peritonitis (FIP).** This viral infection is spread through saliva and feces. Cats become infected through direct contact with a sick cat or by contact with virus-contaminated surfaces such as clothing, feeding bowls, or bedding. Exposure to the virus may cause a transient and mild upper-respiratory illness, associated with sneezing, watery eyes, and nasal discharge. Most cats recover completely. A small percentage, however, develop the symptoms of deadly FIP weeks, months, or even longer after their primary infection. Less than 1 percent of cats seen by veterinarians are symptomatic. The disease rate can be much higher—up to 20 percent—in shelters, catteries, and multicat populations, where there is greater chance for exposure. The typical forms of FIP are described as wet, dry, or a combination of both. In the wet form, the abdomen and/or chest fills with fluid, making it difficult for the cat to breathe. The dry form is characterized by fever, anemia, depression, and weight loss.

- **Feline immunodeficiency virus (FIV).** The FIV virus is regarded as similar to the HIV virus in humans. Over time it causes a deterioration in the ability of the immune system to counteract other viruses and microorganisms in the environment, leaving a cat highly susceptible to secondary infections. Such infections are the major cause of death in cats who are FIV-positive. The virus is spread primarily through bite wounds. Outdoor male cats are the most commonly affected, indoor cats the least. FIV causes a generalized enlargement of the lymph nodes. Poor coat, persistent fever, loss of appetite, and inflammation of the gums, mouth, skin, bladder, and upper-respiratory tract are common signs of an active infection. Researchers say that FIV is a species-specific agent and does not spread to humans.

Examination and laboratory tests are necessary to determine a precise diagnosis for these major viral diseases. Symptoms can be confusing and often relate to other conditions. There is no generally recognized cure for symptomatic animals. Conventional treatments include powerful chemotherapeutic drugs, antibiotics, and steroids, all of which have associated risks of side effects and suppressing the immune system.

Treatments for infections among holistic veterinarians are highly variable. Some emphasize vitamins, others herbs, and still others tailor an individualized program around homeopathic remedies.

HERBS

A WORD OF CAUTION ON ECHINACEA

The popular herb echinacea that we use for colds and flu is a major healing weapon for many holistic veterinarians against viral and bacterial infections. The herb boosts and normalizes the immune system. It works well with chronic infections, ear and respiratory conditions, and sores that won't heal well and for pets who have been on long-term steroids, antibiotics, or any medications that deplete or suppress the immune system.

Veterinarians caution that it should not be used indefinitely. Reports in the herbal literature indicate that continual use over time can overly stimulate and exhaust the immune system. The recommendation is to use it for two or three weeks, stop it for a week or two, and then resume it again if needed. In more severe cases it can be used for three weeks and then stopped for a week.

This approach can be used long-term.

Echinacea does not have a cat-friendly taste. Try to get a nonalcohol tincture in the health food store. If you can find only an alcohol product, you can dilute it to minimize the quantity of the alcohol. Or you can mix it with a food that is highly aromatic, such as tuna oil, or something your cat likes. Cat food has such a strong taste that the animal may not mind the addition.

Echinacea for Respiratory Ills—Pamela Wood-Krzeminski, DVM

Echinacea is particularly useful for upper-respiratory viral conditions often seen in kittens or older cats who have come from shelters. I also recommend vitamin C, in the form of sodium ascorbate crystals. The combination can speed recovery. Unless there is a secondary bacterial infection, indicated by heavy pus, there usually is no need for an antibiotic.

DOSAGE
- **Echinacea:** First add 2 droppers of a standardized extract in 1 ounce of water. Then use a half dropper of that mixture for a cat under five pounds three times a day; for a larger cat, a full dropper.
- **Vitamin C:** 100 milligrams, two to three times a day.

Echinacea Plus Goldenseal—A. Greig Howie, DVM

I recommend using echinacea for general infectious conditions. If the animal is fighting a respiratory or urinary tract infection, I will recommend it along with goldenseal. The combination soothes the lining of the mucous membranes of the body. Goldenseal also has antibiotic activity. Instead of trying to kill off the bugs, try to make the body stronger. These are good agents against both bacteria and viruses.

For me, this approach usually substitutes for antibiotics. But if your veterinarian prescribes antibiotics, you can add these natural remedies to the therapeutic program. They will not interfere, but will help to protect the immune system and also repair some of the damage done by antibiotics.

DOSAGE

- 3 or 4 drops twice a day.

Osha Root for Viruses, Debilitation—Mark Haverkos, DVM

Osha root, known by the Native Americans as bear root, is one of the most powerful herbs on the planet. I recommend this natural agent for any condition diagnosed as viral related or for chronic debilitation, where an animal goes downhill no matter what you do for it. I see good results with it—a general improvement of the whole system. I use this herb often for older cats that are thin and clearly unhealthy. My source of osha root is a tincture made by Winter Sun Trading Co. (520-774-2884).

According to Michael Moore, director of the Southwest School of Botanical Medicine in Albuquerque and an expert on North American herbs, osha root is one of the only botanicals that is truly virucidal—that is, it kills viruses. The herb has long been used by Native Americans, who, according to tradition, first observed bears digging up the root and eating it when ill. Osha root is a blood purifier, immune stimulant, and expectorant (for coughs). It is strong but safe.

Osha smells and tastes like turpentine, a flavor that a cat will surely not like. You need to mix it with tuna oil or a highly aromatic food the animal enjoys. Either that or put the liquid in a capsule and pill the cat.

DOSAGE
- 1 to 5 drops of the tincture once a day. Can be used indefinitely. Try reducing the dosage or discontinue upon improvement, to see if the animal can maintain a higher level of health on its own.

Ashwaganda for Leukemia—Tejinder Sodhi, DVM

For cats diagnosed leukemia positive with anemia, the traditional Indian herb ashwaganda (winter cherry) can be a beneficial addition to treatment. I use a liquid ashwaganda product available through Ayush Herbs (800-925-1371). Research has shown that ashwaganda increases red blood cells. It also increases energy, nourishes the nervous system, and helps the body cope with stress. All these are properties that will help support and stabilize an animal in this situation. Often the appetite will improve after a short while. Ashwaganda will not interact or interfere with any medication.

DOSAGE
- 10 drops per ten pounds of body weight, two or three times a day if possible

HOMEOPATHIC REMEDIES
(See chapter 9 for general dosage guidelines.)

Aconitum for Upper Respiratory—Mark Haverkos, DVM

For sneezing bouts that often plague young cats for weeks, and where the animals aren't spiking a fever and are just slightly off their food, I will use a combination of the homeopathic remedy Aconitum along with the herb pleurisy root. The two should bring improvement within two weeks. Aconite is an excellent remedy for cold-type symptoms. Pleurisy is an expectorant herb that will help the body eliminate pathogens from the mucous membranes. I use the tincture form of pleurisy root, from Winter Sun Trading Co. (520-774-2884). Echinacea can also be used to stimulate the immune system.

DOSAGE

- **Aconitum 30C:** A few drops into the mouth once or twice a day.

- **Pleurisy root:** 1 to 5 drops of the tincture diluted in 1 teaspoon of water, once a day.

Aconitum, Arsenicum, and Gelsemium for Kitty Colds—Joseph Demers, DVM

In the first stage of a cold affecting young cats, you will usually see sneezing with some runny clear discharge from the eyes. In these situations I recommend Aconitum, particularly if the cat is somewhat fearful or jumpy.

Frequent sneezing, coughing, and an increased but still thin discharge indicate the infection is still of a mild nature but somewhat more intense than the first stage. This may now be the second or third day of a cold. Arsenicum album, another homeopathic remedy, is appropriate in this situation. The cat may be rubbing its nose or eyes as if there is a burning sensation or discomfort. It would not be very thirsty and perhaps feel somewhat cold. When you pick up the cat, the ears and the belly may be hot, but the paws and the rest of the body feel cold. This is what we would call a "chilly fever."

For acute head colds with thick discharges, where kittens may be very weak with high fevers, and perhaps shaking legs, the homeopathic remedy Gelsemium works very well.

I have found this simple regime very effective for many kittens. It brings fevers down within a day or two. If the condition does not improve, a different homeopathic remedy is needed. Ideally, consult with a homeopathic veterinarian.

DOSAGE
- Use remedies in pellet form. Crush the pellets in a folded piece of paper or dissolve them in 1 ounce of distilled water, and give the cat half an eyedropperful in the mouth.

- **Aconitum:** Give 2 or 3 pellets of 6C potency, six or seven times a day (every two hours) for two to three days. This usually stops the cold. If not, try a 30C potency two to three times daily.

- **Arsenicum album:** Give 2 or 3 pellets of 6C potency, six or seven times for two to three days. If no decrease in symptoms by the third day, use a 30C potency three times daily for three days.

- **Gelsemium:** Give 2 or 3 pellets of 6C potency, five times daily until the symptoms are better. Use a 30C potency, two or three times a day if no improvement after twenty-four to forty-eight hours.

NUTRITIONAL SUPPLEMENTS

Vaccines No Solution for Leukemia—Jean Hofve, DVM

Many veterinarians recommend vaccinating cats for this viral condition. I do not. There are numerous leukemia virus strains, and each manufacturer's vaccine protects against only a few strains. I have seen cats test positive for leukemia despite being vaccinated regularly for years. Vaccines may protect some cats some of the time. Most veterinary schools do not use the vaccine.

Moreover, the vaccine has been shown to cause a form of cancer called "fibrosarcoma," a connective tissue tumor difficult to treat. The tumor, if removed surgically, can grow back even more vigorously than before. The rabies vaccine has also been implicated as a cause of this cancer, but some evidence suggests that the feline leukemia vaccine is more often the cause. In countries that do not vaccinate for either feline leukemia or rabies, the incidence of fibrosarcoma is zero.

I feel that the risks of the vaccine are worse than the disease itself. I prefer to concentrate on keeping pets healthy though good nutrition and building a healthy immune system. The best defense against leukemia or any other infectious disease is a good immune system.

In my practice I recommend Immuplex, a combination supplement of vitamins, minerals, and glandular tissue formulated to increase the immune system response. The product is made by Standard Process (800-848-5061; sold through veterinarians). This is my favorite supplement for boosting the immune system against any infectious condition where the cat may not be holding its own or in cases of autoimmune diseases where the system is dysfunctional. The supplement helps balance the system.

DOSAGE
- 1 capsule daily.

CHRONIC UPPER-RESPIRATORY INFECTIONS (ALSO KNOWN AS RHINITIS, SINUSITIS, COLDS)

Many cats get colds during their lifetimes, and some will sneeze for weeks. At the first sign of a cold put your animal on vitamin C and antioxidants. Most veterinarians will prescribe antibiotics, but they don't do anything for this condition, which is basically viral in nature. Cats with a chronic condition usually feel okay and are eating well, but they will constantly have a nasal discharge and you will be forever cleaning up snot after them. Often we see this develop in cats out of shelters who have been slammed with the multiple stress of vaccinations and spaying or neutering. Strengthen the immune system and try to prevent the problem from becoming chronic. I recommend vitamin C, in the form of Ester-C, along with Antiox, a grapeseed extract antioxidant for animals, made by Vetri-Science (800-882-9993; sold through veterinarians).

DOSAGE
- **Ester-C:** 200 milligrams daily.
- **Antiox:** Follow label instructions.

FELINE INFECTIOUS PERITONITIS (FIP)

In my practice I find that at least half of the normal cats I do blood-work on test positive for FIP. They have no symptoms. Their immune systems are dealing with the virus.

Kittens will sometimes develop a short-lived diarrhea caused by the corona virus, the same virus associated with FIP. However, if a cat comes down with FIP symptoms, such as the bloated abdomen due to an abnormal fluid buildup, this is serious. I regard that as a 100 percent failure of the immune system.

If a cat in your household has died of FIP, and you have other cats, don't panic. It is not a death sentence for the other animals. It is extremely unlikely that the other cats will be affected. They have probably already been dealing with it effectively on their own. If tested, they will very likely be positive, but this is to be expected. A major study done in England involving hundreds of cats indicated there was an extremely low incidence of transmission from one cat to another. My advice is to keep the immune systems strong with a good diet, vitamin C, and antioxidants (refer to dosage under upper-respiratory conditions on the previous page). Don't stress the cats. This would not be the time for vaccinations, dentistry, or going on vacation. They need your support.

Fighting Viruses with Vitamin C—Wendell Belfield, DVM

For twenty-five years I have successfully used a nutritional supplement with vitamin C and other vitamin and mineral nutrients to turn virus-positive cats negative. This immune-boosting formula, called Mega-C Plus (available from Orthomolecular Specialties at 408-227-9334), has never failed and to date has helped hundreds of cats found to be carriers of feline leukemia (FeLV), feline infectious peritonitis (FIP), and feline immunodeficiency (FIV) viruses. The supplement comes in powder form and is mixed into the food. Use enough of the supplement so that the animal is receiving the equivalent of 750 milligrams of vitamin C daily. In addition, be sure the animal is getting at least 750 IU of vitamin A and 100 IU of vitamin E.

The amount of time required to turn a cat from positive to negative is variable and depends on the animal. I have seen this occur in as little as nine weeks and as long as three years. An older animal will tend to take longer, but you will start to see a healthier cat as the supplement builds up the body.

Give the supplement long-term, particularly if a cat has weakened immunity that is genetically linked or may be subjected to stress in the environment. Cats can return to virus-positive status and an immune-weakened state, leaving them susceptible to disease.

Keep in mind that I am speaking of animals who are not symptomatic. If a cat has symptoms of viral disease and is not eating, be sure to see a veterinarian.

Mega-C Plus is a highly effective preventive supplement for all these viral conditions. Cattery operators have been using it successfully for years. When queens are supplemented during pregnancy and lactation, the kittens develop optimum immunity through the placenta and milk. Soon after birth they themselves begin receiving the supplement. This simple practice has helped to dramatically reduce the incidence of upper-respiratory disease among the kittens.

The product is available in liquid form for kittens and as a powder for weaned and older animals.

DOSAGE
• Follow label instructions.

MIXED AND MISCELLANEOUS APPROACHES

Helping Susceptible Animals—Donna Starita Mehan, DVM

For animals prone to chronic infections, I use a combination of several nutritional supplements and herbs that can abort or significantly shorten the duration of infectious episodes. The combination consists of a good multi-vitamin/mineral formula for pets, colloidal silver, Spectra Probiotic, and EHB. Spectra is a multistrain beneficial bacteria product that replenishes the good bacteria that the body needs. EHB is a supplement containing echinacea, goldenseal, and barberry, important herbal immune boosters. Spectra and EHB are made by NF Formulas (800-547-4891).

If a herpes virus is involved, I will add the amino acid lysine. Herpes is usually involved in chronic bladder, eye, upper-respiratory, and throat infections and inflammatory conditions of the gums such as stomatitis.

DOSAGE

- **Multi-vitamin/mineral formula:** Follow label instructions.

- **Colloidal silver:** 2 to 10 drops twice daily. Use product with 500 parts per million of silver.

- **Spectra:** 1/4 capsule.

- **EHB:** 1/4 capsule twice daily.

- **Lysine:** 250 milligrams twice daily for the average-size cat.

The Hormonal Connection—Alfred Plechner, DVM

I treat many sick cats that have outright symptoms of FeLV, FIP, and FIV. I use a combination of approaches that includes a multi-vitamin/mineral supplement, digestive enzymes, and hormonal replacement. The results are excellent. Seventy percent of them with FIV and FIP will live and be normally healthy. For FeLV, the results are even better, about 85 percent.

It is critical that these animals eat food that is not offensive to them (see Plechner's comment in food allergy section). If you give them food that they are individually allergic to, you run a high risk of triggering autoimmune turmoil in their bodies. In my experience I have found these animals are often hormonally deficient. They have genetically flawed and imbalanced hormones that generate wild immune responses. Their white blood cells chase down and kill the viruses, then stampede out of control and kill the cat.

Often chemotherapeutic agents are used to treat these conditions. Chemo ravages the immune system. Then you have two major systems—the hormonal and the immune—that are ravaged. Imagine what happens to the cat.

For all these cases I use a special blood test available to veterinarians (see chapter 15 on when nothing seems to work) that measures key hormonal and immune activity. The test enables me to calibrate a proper hormonal replacement therapy that goes along with good nutrition and supplements to restore these cats to health. In catteries or multicat households, if any animals test positive for any of these infections, I highly recommend having the animals tested. If the results are normal, I find that cats tend not to develop symptoms. If results are not normal, your veterinarian can help prevent an outbreak by correcting the existing imbalance with the proper hormonal replacement.

With hormonal and immune imbalances, animals tend to be intolerant to many foods and develop a secondary set of food allergy-related symptoms. Supplementation with digestive enzymes provides an essential therapeutic benefit for these animals. The enzymes aid in breaking down and utilizing food.

⩗ Kidney Failure ⩔

Kidney disease is the second leading cause of disease-related feline death. Among older cats, it is the number one cause. The body's two kidneys are critical to health. They remove wastes from the blood and combine them with water for their journey out the urinary tract. Usually the disease involves scarred, inflamed, and shrunken organs that progressively weaken the critical filtering activity. If kidneys cannot effectively eliminate wastes, internal poisoning (uremia) develops, a buildup of toxicity that can be fatal.

Signs of kidney failure include the following:

- Increased thirst and urination, what one veterinarian describes as "the drink a lot, pee a lot syndrome."
- Decreased appetite.
- Weight loss and wasting.
- Occasional vomiting.
- Bad breath. Also a smell of urine on the skin.
- Dull coat, loss of hair, heavy shedding.

Annual checkups, including bloodwork, can help alert your veterinarian to a developing kidney problem. The outward signs above may not become apparent until the disease is well advanced. Experts say they do not typically occur until more than 70 percent of kidney function is lost.

When the kidneys begin to give out, you will notice a cat drinking and urinating more than usual. This could be the sign of other problems, such as diabetes, so it is important to get a veterinarian's diagnosis.

Despite a cat's increasing drinking, kidney failure also produces dehydration in the body. The organs are no longer effectively conserving water. "If you pinch the skin at the shoulder and it settles back very slowly, that's a good sign of dehydration and a kidney problem," says Ron Carsten, DVM. "Normally, the skin would spring right back. Look also at the gums. Instead of their normal moist condition, they will look dry and tacky."

Holistic veterinarians blame kidney disease primarily on three culprits:

1. Genetically weak kidneys.

2. Exposure to excess toxins such as insecticides and chemically treated drinking water.

3. Poor diet; a lifetime of processing poor protein and filtering out chemical additives.

Holistic veterinarians say that because the quality of pet food is often so nutritionally poor, they now see kidney problems among younger animals than they used to years ago. The quality, they say, just doesn't create or maintain healthy organs, kidneys included.

Conventional veterinary medicine offers little hope for animals with advanced disease. Once a diagnosis is made, your veterinarian will recommend fluid therapy to correct dehydration and flush the body of wastes, thus reducing the risk of internal poisoning. Such therapy may be essential to reduce the risk of internal poisoning. Most veterinarians will also prescribe medication to reduce inflammation and pain and increase appetite. They may also prescribe a prescription diet low in protein. The kidneys remove the waste products left after the body breaks down protein, so the rationale is that a diet lower in protein takes strain off the kidneys.

SPECIAL FOODS AND DIET

Consider the Raw Meat Solution—Bill Pollak, DVM

I am a big believer of feeding a large amount of raw meat to cats, even if they have kidney problems. Normally, cats with kidney disease are put on restricted, low-protein diets. The protein in commercial food is of such poor quality that it acts in the body as a direct toxin and irritant to the kidneys. So if you reduce the level of such protein the animal will benefit, but improvement tends to be only of a transient nature, and then the system falls unmistakably apart. The point is not the quantity of the protein. The issue is the quality. The standard restricted diets still contain poor-quality protein sources. Such food simply does not contain enough vitality, freshness, and variety to generate real, long-lasting health. Cats with very poor blood tests involving the kidneys will often improve dramatically on raw meat. It's the freshness and naturalness of this most appropriate food source for cats—raw meat—that drives the healing process. The vitality in the meat is transferred to the weakened organ for effective repair.

Diet and Natural Remedies—Robert Goldstein, VMD

Holistic therapies can help a good deal. Specific natural remedies and proper nutrients nourish the kidneys and strengthen the entire body's efficiency.

I prefer a home-cooked kidney diet to the prescription diets, which often contain by-products and wastes from the human food industry. I feel these diets tax the kidneys. As an alternative, I developed a recipe that may be served alone or mixed with any natural, low-protein food. It meets all the needs of a kidney patient.

THE ALTERNATIVE KIDNEY DIET
- 1 cup brown rice or millet
- 3 cups filtered or distilled water
- 2 egg yolks (organic, if possible)
- 1/2 cup boneless, skinless chicken, cubed (preferably hormone and antibiotic free)
- 2 tablespoons minced parsley
- 2 tablespoons grated asparagus
- 1 tablespoon sesame oil (unrefined)

Multi-vitamin/mineral (Daily Health Nuggets, from Earth Animal at 800-711-2292, or Maximum Protection Formula, from Dr. Goodpet at 800-222-9932). Follow label instructions.

Directions: Cook rice or millet well with 2 1/2 cups of water for about 45 minutes. With remaining water, cook chicken slightly for 5 minutes. Add finely chopped raw vegetables, eggs, and oil to cooked grain. The parsley and asparagus act as gentle diuretics, helping the kidneys flush out impurities. If the eggs are organic, add them raw. If not organic, soft boil them first. Add supplement to cooled mixture. If your animal has a poor appetite, flavor the mixture with raw, organic liver or organic fat-free yogurt (2 teaspoons). As a full meal, feed 1/4 to 1/2 cup. As a topping over a natural-base senior-type food, reduce the amount of commercial food by the amount of "topper" recipe added.

I also recommend the following nutritional and natural remedies, which can extend and improve the day-to-day quality of your animal's life. When trying this program, watch your animal's appetite closely. That's a good way to tell if wastes are increasing in the blood. If the appetite weakens, even slightly, see your veterinarian at once.

To create an individually tailored nutritional and remedy program for patients with kidney failure and other serious, life-threatening conditions, I use a special test I developed years ago. The test is called the Bio-Nutritional Analysis and is available to veterinarians at 800-670-0830 (for more details see chapter 15).

Remedies and Dosage

- **Renatrate,** an extract of kidney tissue, made by Progressive Laboratories (800-527-9512). 1/2 tablet twice daily.

- **Renal Drops,** a combination homeopathic remedy to help rebuild kidneys, made by Professional Health Products (800-929-4133); ask your veterinarian to order it for you. Give 3 to 5 drops twice daily, apart from food.

- **Solidago, Inflammation, and Exhaustion,** three homeopathic remedies in tablet form made by BHI Laboratories (800-621-7644) and available through health food stores or pharmacies. Dissolve 6 tablets of each remedy in a 2-ounce glass eyedropper bottle filled with distilled water. Shake well. Give 1/3 of a dropper three times daily apart from food. Store in refrigerator after mixing.

Homemade Food Is Best—Jean Hofve, DVM

I have been increasingly alarmed by the sight of younger and younger cats with failing kidneys. Recently I saw a 2 1/2-year-old cat who died of kidney failure.

The most beneficial measure you can do is to give your cat subcutaneous fluids. This helps flush toxins out of the bloodstream for animals who cannot drink enough to compensate for the loss of water due to failing kidneys. Ask your veterinarian to show you how to do it. It is very simple.

Options are limited when this condition is advanced. We can't create new kidney cells when scar tissue has already formed. But homeopathy, herbs, Bach flowers, or acupuncture may make your cat feel better. For an individualized program, consult with a holistic veterinarian.

I recommend a high-moisture diet to keep up the cat's fluid levels. Do not feed dry food alone. Kidney problems are accelerated by a diet of dry food that too many people feed their animals.

You may have heard that restricting protein is recommended for cats in kidney failure. According to Martin Fettman, DVM, of the Colorado State University's School of Veterinary Medicine, restricted protein diets have no effect on the development or progression of renal disease and only questionable effects on symptoms. Furthermore, cats usually don't like the prescription diets and often won't eat them. It you have ever looked at this food, you'll know why. It looks and smells horrible! It is more important that a sick cat eats, so give it what it likes in order to maintain weight and body condition. The best thing is a home-prepared diet.

To supplement the diet, I use Renafood, a nutritional supplement made by Standard Process (800-848-5061; sold through veterinarians). It contains organ extracts and natural enzymes designed to detoxify and support the kidneys.

DOSAGE
• 1 to 2 tablets a day. Crush tabs and add to food.

⚜ Lack of Appetite ⚜

Lack of appetite is a common warning sign for many different illnesses affecting cats and should be brought to a veterinarian's attention. Call your veterinarian if the following occurs, particularly if your cat is an older or obese animal:

- It refuses food or takes only a few nibbles for more than two meals.
- It shows signs of illness such as lethargy, decreased grooming, vomiting, or abnormal stool.

A quick response on your part may help prevent the rapid onset of an acute and deadly liver condition. Healthy cats will occasionally fast for a day or so. If your cat appears strong and healthy, has no symptoms of illness, and ignores food now and then, don't mind. Regard it as a natural act of rest and purification by an animal attuned to its biological needs.

⚜ Liver Disease ⚜

The liver is the body's chemical factory, a central organ that masterminds the processing and utilization of the carbohydrates, fats, and proteins that are eaten as well as the removal of toxic substances. When its complex mechanisms go wrong, people and animals alike suffer in many ways.

Degeneration of the liver frequently affects older cats and can cause repercussions throughout the body. Many signs of a failing liver are easily confused with, or associated with, many other medical problems, so a diagnosis is needed. Common signs include vomiting, lethargy and tiring easily, decreased appetite, irritability, and jaundice. Regular checkups, including bloodwork, can help spot liver trouble at an early date.

Cats, particularly obese animals, are prone to a peculiar and life-threatening disorder called "hepatic lipidosis"—or fatty liver syndrome. It typically occurs after an animal has not been eating for a period of time. The lack of food causes the body to break down fat stores to supply needed energy. A flood of fat enters the liver for processing and clogs the organ, virtually putting it out of commission. The animal now has no appetite and is at high risk of dying from liver failure. Treatment usually requires forced feeding through a tube.

HERBS

Milk Thistle Protects the Liver—A. Greig Howie, DVM

For any liver condition—hepatitis, fatty liver, chronic liver disease, inflammation of the bile ducts—don't hesitate to use milk thistle. This herb has amazing healing effects and actually regenerates the liver.

You can add milk thistle to any treatment program, and it may very well be the only thing that will help. I don't know of any drug we veterinarians have that will regenerate the liver, but milk thistle will definitely do it. You will see big improvement with this herb. Your veterinarian will gauge improvement by doing standard liver enzyme tests, and I am sure that he or she will be surprised, as I was in the beginning, at how well this herb improves the status of the liver. This is a very organ-specific herb. Once the enzyme level normalizes you can stop the herb.

Many studies have validated milk thistle's protective effect against poison. It works protectively and also repairs the liver from exposure to poisons.

If the animal is on any medication that puts a particular burden on the liver, use milk thistle daily. Heartworm medication, for instance, is hard on the liver. I will start the animal on milk thistle prior to the medication so it protects the liver against the chemicals that kill the heartworms. Some of the cancer drugs are toxic to the liver, and again, milk thistle can offer protection.

If an animal has a damaged liver or a history of liver problems, I suggest giving milk thistle daily for a week each month.

More on Milk Thistle—Pamela Wood-Krzeminski, DVM

Along with any other therapy, I always recommend milk thistle to help heal the liver. I have had good success with the milk thistle

(*Silymarin*) extract from Twin Labs, available in health food stores. One way to get a cat to take it is to empty the contents into a palatable food, such as one of the meaty baby foods.

DOSAGE
- 1 capsule daily.

Milk Thistle Plus Homeopathics—Maria Glinski, DVM

I have seen excellent results for liver conditions by adding two natural remedies:

- Milk thistle, in the form of a liquid, glycerin-based product from Gaia Herbs (800-831-7780), available at health food stores. Give 10 drops twice a day.

- Liver Liquessence, a homeopathic combination remedy from Professional Health Products (800-929-4133, sold through health professionals only). The formula includes lycopodium, hydrastis, taraxacum, chelidonium, and liver gland. Give 2 drops on the tongue four times daily during the first month, decreasing to two times for three months or until liver blood values are normal. For best results, administer in a clean mouth. You want the drops to be absorbed by the mucous membranes.

Milk Thistle and Glutamine—Ron Carsten, DVM

I have found that a majority of liver problems are closely linked to a digestive tract that is not functioning as well as it should. To help against this, I recommend the amino acid glutamine, which is a primary energy source for intestinal cells, along with milk thistle.

This simple supplement program can substantially enhance any treatment your veterinarian has prescribed. Cats often start to look and eat better and become more active. Give supplements with meals.

DOSAGE
- **Milk thistle:** 250 milligrams once a day.
- **Glutamine:** 500 milligrams twice.

Ayurvedic Herbs for the Liver—Tejinder Sodhi, DVM

I have had excellent results with an Ayurvedic herbal combination from India called Livit-2, prepared by Ayush Herbs (800-925-1371).

The product is available in liquid form for cats. The formula contains multiple herbs, among them kutli (*Picrorhiza kurroa*), which has been shown by research to detoxify the liver, eliminate excess or impure bile, and purify the blood; and amla (*Emblica officinalis*), which helps rejuvenate the immune system and increase the red blood cell count. Amla is the richest source of vitamin C among all fruits and also contains phytochemicals recognized for antioxidant properties and immune enhancement.

I recommend this formula when blood tests reveal elevated liver enzymes, a sign of trouble in the liver that could indicate such problems as acute hepatitis, congestion, or a buildup of toxicity from medication. Livit-2 protects, nourishes, and detoxifies the liver. I believe it is more effective than milk thistle alone. Within two to three weeks animals usually feel better, although it will often take longer for tests to show a normalization of the liver enzymes. Blood tests done a month after starting on the product usually show a decrease toward normalization of the enzyme levels. After another two months there is typically a dramatic drop.

This product is very protective against the toxicity of drugs when animals undergo chemotherapy. We see improved appetite, more energy, less vomiting, and, in general, fewer problems related to the medication. Livit-2 supports any therapy and medication by fortifying and protecting the liver.

DOSAGE
• 10 drops twice daily per ten pounds. Use the formula for at least three months or until liver enzymes normalize, or longterm while the animal is taking strong medication such as phenobarbital for epilepsy or chemotherapeutic drugs.

Herbal, Glandular, and Mineral Formula—Jean Hofve, DVM

In addition to standard therapy, I recommend Livaplex, a glandular supplement made by Standard Process (800-848-5061; sold through veterinarians). The product contains liver extracts, herbs, and minerals and provides excellent detoxifying and general support for a cat on a therapeutic program. Your veterinarian may not be familiar with this product, but it is definitely worth using.

Dosage
• 1 tablet a day mixed with food.

◢ **Motion Sickness** ◣

To eliminate the anxiety and motion sickness associated with transporting animals, Rescue Remedy, a popular flower essence (see chapter 10), is often recommended, either by itself or in combination with other remedies.

As a general rule, don't feed animals before traveling. They may throw up during the trip. If you are going on an extended car ride, feed only at night when you arrive at your destination. You can offer water on stops, but chances are cats won't drink.

Calm with Rescue Remedy—Pamela Wood-Krzeminski, DVM

I've had good success with Rescue Remedy, a liquid product available in health food stores. You can give it directly in the mouth straight, add to the drinking water, or put a couple of drops on the cat's ears and rub gently into the skin.

Dosage
• Give before departure and use as often as needed—every half hour or couple of hours to keep animal calm.

Rescue Remedy Plus Elm, Walnut—Jean Hofve, DVM

The combination of Rescue Remedy plus Elm and Walnut, all flower essences, works excellently for traveling or moving with a cat. Purchase the individual bottles of flower remedies at a health food store, then combine them in the following manner: Put 2 drops from each bottle into a fresh, clean 1-ounce bottle filled with spring water. This bottle then becomes the remedy you will dispense.

If you are packing for weeks before a move, cats will be very aware of the activity and may become anxious. To allay the anxiety, put the combination of flower essences in a spray bottle and spray around in the rooms where you are packing. It will help infuse calmness into the environment—for both the animals and the people involved.

DOSAGE
- Start administering, if possible, at least several days beforehand and preferably two weeks before if you are making a major move.

Homeopathics for a Smooth Ride—Roger DeHaan, DVM

I like CalmStress, a homeopathic liquid formula from Dr. Goodpet (800-222-9932) that works quite well for motion sickness and stress. I often mix CalmStress and Rescue Remedy. The combination appears to be even more effective than either one individually.

DOSAGE
- Use either product singly and follow label instructions. Or, to combine the two, add 6 drops of Rescue Remedy to a bottle of CalmStress. Shake well. Whether combined or singly, start remedy a day or two before departure on an extended automobile or air journey. Add to animal's drinking water as well as giving directly in the mouth several times a day. Give remedy two hours before, one hour before, and just prior to getting into the car. One reason for starting ahead of time is that many animals become anxious when they sense an upcoming trip. Some animals pick up readily on a "traveling vibe." During an extended ride in the automobile, giving the remedy orally every two to four hours is helpful.

⬇ Obesity ⬇

Cats, like people, have their weight problems. Stats on cats suggest that a quarter of the feline population may be overweight. In a 1989 study of two thousand cats treated at thirty-one clinics, Cornell University researchers ranked 20 percent of the animals as heavy and 5 percent as obese. Then, in a follow-up 1997 study, the investigators determined that the heavier cats were at much higher risk of developing health problems than optimum weight felines. Fat cats were:

- 4 1/2 times more likely to have diabetes.
- 3 times more likely to suffer from lameness and 7 times more likely to need veterinary care for lameness related to arthritis and muscle injuries.
- 3 times more likely to need treatment for nonallergic skin problems.
- twice as likely to die before the age of twelve.

Which cats become "fat cats"? The researchers made these conclusions from the data:

- Apartment cats are twice as likely as outdoor cats or animals living in larger dwellings.
- Neutered cats are 3.4 times more likely than non-neutered animals.
- Inactive cats that get no exercise are 16 times more likely.

One interesting finding was that many cats put on the extra weight early in life. By two years of age nearly 20 percent of the surveyed cats were already too heavy.

Pet owners tend to overfeed animals, and their systems simply cannot process the volume adequately. Too many calories go in. Usually not enough go out in the form of exercise. Similar to humans, again. Too many calorie-rich snacks? Cut them out.

Dry pet food has three times the calories as canned food. If you have a heavier animal, start giving it more wet food and less dry. Interestingly, the Cornell researchers found that some of the so-called prescription diets are even more likely to contribute to heaviness because they contain more calories than regular food.

A cat won't jog with you. It may walk with you. But for sure you need to bring more exercise opportunities into its life. Stock the premises with some pet toys that will stimulate your cat into action. Interactive exercises—involving something as simple as a toy dangling on the end of a string—are good for the cat's health and waistline and for bonding.

Obesity is often, but not always, a simple problem of too many calories and not enough activity. In the same household with two cats of the same breed and age eating the same amount of excess food, one might become overweight and the other not—just like humans.

Susan G. Wynn, DVM, notes that "placid, relaxed animals may gain weight more easily than pets with a lot of nervous energy. Genetic makeup also plays a large role, and some pets are simply going to lose and maintain their weight better than others."

Veterinarians treat obesity individually because it can often involve a complex metabolic problem such as an imbalance in the digestive-hormonal relationship that is unique in each case. Disorders of the adrenal and thyroid glands, as well as overmedication with steroids, may be associated with weight gain.

Obesity is a serious medical and nutritional problem and should be brought to your veterinarian's attention.

HOW TO TELL IF YOUR CAT IS TOO HEAVY

- You can't feel the ribs easily.
- There is more than just a light cover of fat under the skin.
- The stomach is loose and flabby and not tucked up.

FOOD AND SPECIAL DIETS

More Quality, Less Quantity—William Pollak, DVM

Commercial pet food will often make animals overweight and give them a dull, doughy, edematous appearance. This is generally food designed not with quality, but with taste in mind. If your animal eats it, you think it must be good. It doesn't mean that at all. It just means that the manufacturer has succeeded in putting flavors into the food that basically cover up the poor quality of the ingredients, or a food your pet would not eat if it were not for the addictive agents that are included. Your animal eats more to take more nutrition into its body. That means more calories. Your overweight animal is essentially overfed and undernourished. Animals who eat a more natural diet, with raw food, generally tend to eat less. That's because the food is higher in nutrient quality. The animal actually gets more nutrition from less food. It's a simple concept: quality vs. quantity. On a natural diet, after eating a commercial diet, your animal loses weight, its body become more dense. You see the muscles and its natural confirmation. You see more health and vitality.

Two Diets for Heavyweights—Edmund Dorosz, DVM

If your cat has no medical problem that may be causing the excess weight, there are a number of simple measures you can follow to promote a loss of body fat while conserving lean muscle tissue.

Feed less—up to 30 percent less—and more often. Small, frequent portions can be very effective. A teaspoon of food every three or four hours is sufficient. This allows the stomach to shrink so that hunger is easily satisfied. A teaspoon of these foods given often will trim down a cat: yogurt, cottage cheese, sour cream, sardines, turkey, beef, lamb, chicken, duck, hamburger, liver, fish, cooked egg, or kidney. A raw egg is okay also if you use the whole egg.

And provide more exercise and play. Make sure that includes mental exercise. Without any stimulation, indoor cats can become lazy and depressed and just lie about and eat. Cats need to use their brain, just as they did when they were hunting in the wilds. If you have indoor cats, be sure to provide enough mental stimulation with some of the many pet toys available on the market.

The following two recipes are excellent for weight loss.

Low-Fat Diet

If your cat will eat vegetables, this recipe provides balanced proteins, vitamins, and minerals. Here I use bulk to give a feeling of fullness.

> *Ingredients*
> 4 ounces lean ground beef
> 1/2 cup dry cottage cheese
> 2 cups cooked carrots
> 2 cups green beans
> 1 teaspoon bone meal
> 1/2 teaspoon garlic powder or catnip

> *Directions:* Cook beef; drain fat. Mix with other ingredients. Sprinkle with garlic or catnip. Feeds fifteen-pound cat for three days.

Beef Tongue

This is a tasty low-calorie, high-fiber diet.

> 1 pound diced beef tongue
> 2 sliced carrots
> 2 celery stalks, with leaves chopped
> 1 cup low-sodium tomato juice

1 cup water
1 teaspoon bone meal
1 teaspoon catnip
2 teaspoons cornstarch
2 tablespoons water
3 teaspoons chopped parsley

Directions: Mix first seven ingredients in a blender and simmer for 1 hour. Mix cornstarch with 2 tablespoons of water and add slowly to tongue mixture. Stir and cook until thickened. Add parsley. Let cool. Feeds a fifteen- to eighteen-pound cat for four days.

No Restricted Diets for Cats—Jean Hofve, DVM

A client recently brought in a twenty-six-pound cat—the fattest cat I ever saw. I asked the owner what he fed the animal.

"Only a quarter cup of dry food a day," he answered.

"Nothing else?" I asked.

"Nothing," he said, "except for fifteen or so of those Pounce cat treats."

I told the owner he could help his cat lose weight by stopping the treats and not leaving the cat's food out. I don't think this advice was what he wanted to hear, because he never returned.

Leaving food out all day can cause fat cats. If I had nothing to do all day but consume food and treats, then I, too, would put on weight. Many cats eat excessively out of boredom or for comfort, and not for hunger, or, as in this case, they eat as a result of an owner's misguided care.

I don't recommend a restrictive diet; that could cause liver problems. If you restrict the diet too much, you could kill the animal. Overweight cats have very sensitive livers. Just change the feeding pattern. Add more wet food. Dry food is calorically dense. You can eat a lot of it before you get filled. Wet food fills them up, is mostly water, and is better for them anyway, and then they eat less of the dry food. Leave the food out for a half hour, or one hour maximum, and then remove it. Throw away leftover wet food or meat.

MIXED AND MISCELLANEOUS APPROACHES

The Second Cat Solution—Michele Yasson, DVM

Today's pets often lead solitary and sedentary lives cooped up in small apartments with owners away working much of the day. For many such animals, weight gain is a natural result of this unnatural existence. For those fat cats stuck inside, try the second cat solution—bring in a playmate.

A second animal will stimulate activity and movement and is often curative for obesity. This approach can work for animals who are depressed and don't eat well. A little competition at the dinner plate really works. Be sure to introduce the animals correctly. For cats who are generally more solitary as adults, it is important to get the "right match." Usually I recommend the opposite gender. If you have a quiet cat, you don't want to bring in a rambunctious animal.

You may want to let the cats meet with a barrier between them or keep the new one in a room by itself for a while, with its own litter and own food. Let them both get used to the idea that this is home and this is where another cat is living. If they suddenly meet face-to-face, it could possibly be very threatening, particularly for the first cat.

Situations obviously will vary. You can put them together as soon as they can get along without hissing or growling.

Sometimes animals will bond immediately. Once a woman brought two cats to board with me for a week. I asked if she would like us to put the animals together in a large cage.

"No," she said, "the older cat hates the younger cat."

So we put them in adjoining cages with a wall between them. Outside the cage, at the front end next to the wall, we tied a toy for the young cat to play with. After a short time, both were playing with the toy through the cage and soon were touching paws and playing with each other even though they couldn't see each other. After the animals returned home, the woman called to say they had become good friends. Be creative. Even something as simple as a toy can sometimes bring animals together.

A variation on this theme is day care for pets. If you and a friend have cats, and both animals are alone during the day, you might want to arrange to have the animals spend time together during the work week. I have many clients who do this. They have found other people in their buildings, or nearby, with lone animals and arranged day care "matches" that bring animal play partners together and provide for some calorie-expending opportunities for the animals.

⇘ Old Age ⇙

Domestic cats live on the average from twelve to fifteen years, although many feline Methuselahs push on for twenty or more.

Veterinarians recommend regular checkups once or more a year, so that any early signs of disease can be detected and the appropriate health care strategies worked out. As they age you may see such typical signs as reduced activity and longer sleeping hours, a graying muzzle, thinning hair coat, looser skin, stiff joints or even lameness, and less tolerance to stress and changes in the routine.

If your older cat is losing weight, and drinks and urinates more than usual, be sure to see a veterinarian at once. These are signs of possible diabetes, kidney failure, or hyperthyroidism. Don't wait. These are all potential time bombs. The longer you wait, the more an organ declines or a disease advances, and the harder it becomes for a veterinarian to treat. There are fewer options. When problems are addressed earlier, they are easier to fight.

My advice is to reduce the amount of protein you feed an older animal. Be alert to changes in food intake, weight, the amount that animals drink, pee, and poop. If all these things stay the same, fine. If any changes occur, check them out.

Providing an optimum diet is one major way to ensure a maximum life span with a good quality of life even as your pet ages and its vital organs lose their youthful efficiency. Diet is critical. Many veterinarians say that middle-aged animals often appear much older than their chronological ages because of weakened organs due to poor diet.

NUTRITIONAL SUPPLEMENTS

Multiple Vitamin/Mineral—Carvel Tiekert, DVM

I often supplement older animals with a good multi-vitamin/mineral, because as they get older they do not absorb the nutrients from their food as efficiently as when they were younger. In addition, their nutritional needs may be higher.

Whole-Food Supplements—Roger DeHaan, DVM

I recommend two whole-food pet supplements that work very well to reenergize older animals and build up their health. Either one is excellent. If an animal doesn't like the taste of one, try the other. Follow label instructions for both products.

1. Vita-Dreams Daily Greens, from Halo (800-426-4256), contains vitamins, minerals, amino acids, chlorophyll, barley and alfalfa juice, bee pollen, bee propolis, and royal jelly.

2. Missing Link, from Designing Health Inc. (800-774-7387). It contains enzymes, fatty acids, fiber, beneficial bacteria, vitamins, trace minerals, and health-boosting compounds from plants.

Digestive Enzymes—Jean Hofve, DVM

Supplementation with a good plant-based digestive enzyme product for pets is a simple and effective preventive measure that can head off pancreas problems and reduce the potential for food allergies.

Vitamin E—Wendell Belfield, DVM

Vitamin E has worked reliably for me over the years to help revitalize aging animals. Studies show that older animals need more of this important antioxidant vitamin in order to slow down the oxidative deterioration of tissue associated with aging. Research also shows that vitamin E improves circulation, the immune system, endurance, stamina, libido, and skin.

The first cat I ever put on vitamin E many years ago was Jake, a ten-year-old orange tabby who was being harassed by neighborhood cats, in particular two younger, virile toms. Within a few weeks the owner called to tell me that her timid, decrepit cat had been transformed into a tiger on 100 IU of vitamin E daily.

"He fights back now and wins," she told me, "and what's more, he is showing renewed interest in females." A few months later the woman called to say that Jake had sired a litter. We decided to test the influence of the vitamin by stopping it for a short while. Within a few weeks Jake had regressed. We restarted the vitamin, and in two weeks the new Jake returned—full of vim and vigor.

FOOD AND SPECIAL DIETS

Vegetables—Norman C. Ralston, DVM

It is very helpful if you can get cats to start eating fresh vegetables. Vegetables clean up the gut and act like a broom, sweeping out toxins. Don't overcook the vegetables, just steam or cook them lightly.

MIXED AND MISCELLANEOUS APPROACHES

Herbal/Flower Essence Pick-Me-Up—Shannon Hines, DVM

As a pick-me-up and all-around tonic, I recommend Senior Support for Cats, a liquid combination of herbs and flower essences made by Tasha's Herbs (800-315-0142). This product promotes health, appetite, and energy. It contains hawthorn berry, nettles, alfalfa, oat-flowers, chamomile, dandelion root and leaf, kelp, and, for palatability plus nutrition, cod liver oil, vitamin E, and lecithin.

DOSAGE
- Follow label instructions.

⤳ Parasites ⤳

Feline intestines are playgrounds for parasites. As many as 45 percent of cats are estimated to have various degrees of worm and protozoan infections. Depending on the severity of the problem, animals may lose their appetite, experience vomiting and diarrhea, and become more susceptible to illnesses. You can help prevent your cats from becoming a victim of common parasites by maintaining good flea control as well as sanitation practices such as cleaning the litter box regularly and removing stool daily.

GIARDIA

Herbs for Relief—Tejinder Sodhi, DVM

Giardia is a common protozoan parasite that reproduces in the intestines of animals and causes diarrhea. Infections are typically picked up from feces, exposure to infected animals, or contaminated water. The problem is more prevalent in catteries and multicat households. Giardia is usually treated with Flagyl (metronidazole), an antiparasitic drug that unfortunately has many side effects. Among other things, it affects balance and the ability to walk.

I have successfully used a combination of two herbal formulas. One is called AP Mag, made by Ayush Herbs (800-925-1371), and includes bael fruit, bitter melon, China berries, berberis, and basil leaf. The other formula is DGL Plus, from Pure Encapsulations (800-753-2277), with licorice root and unripe plantain.

Start with DGL Plus and AP Mag. Use DGL Plus for about two to three weeks to firm up the stool and calm the intestine. AP Mag is used for two to three months or as long as it takes to resolve the condition. If an animal goes through cycles of improvement and relapse, I then strengthen the program with another Ayush product called Neem Plus, an Ayurvedic liquid formula containing neem and several potent antiparasitic herbs.

This herbal program can be discontinued once repeated testing of the feces is negative for parasites and there is a complete resolution of symptoms.

Dosage

- **DGL Plus:** 1 capsule twice daily. Open capsule and mix well into food. It has a bland taste and is well tolerated by cats.

- **AP Mag:** 1 capsule twice daily. This capsule is rather large for a cat. The contents should be be put into smaller capsules. Cats won't like the taste. You will have to pill the cat. Use fish oil or butter to lubricate capsules to make swallowing easier.

- **Neem Plus:** Cats up to ten pounds, 10 drops twice daily; cats up to twenty pounds, 20 drops twice daily.

WORMS

ABOUT WORMING TREATMENT AND MEDICATION

If you suspect your cat has worms, or you live in an area with a known worm problem, it is best to work closely with your veterinarian to develop a prevention, diagnosis, or treatment strategy. Ideally, have your cat examined twice annually for worms. Internal parasites can cause many problems in the intestinal tract and elsewhere in the body.

Many holistic veterinarians advocate the chemical dewormers to quickly rid an animal of an infestation. They regard the new generation of worm medicines available to veterinarians as safer, less toxic, and more effective than previous products.

Holistic practitioners often recommend using the best of both worlds—a combination of chemical dewormers and natural approaches. "Worms tend to be hard to treat naturally," explains Michele Yasson, DVM. "We work with conventional medications to clear out the problem first and then focus on building up the health of the animal with natural means."

Be wary of store-bought chemical dewormers, the veterinarians advise. It is best to check with your veterinarian before using one. "They are generally older products and may contain very potent chemicals, including toluene, an organophosphate," warns Pamela Wood-Krzeminski, DVM. "I have seen animals die of liver failure on this. Other dewormers may be purgatives that get rid of the worms but cause cramps for twelve hours. They work but are too harsh."

HOOKWORMS

These bloodsucking parasites cause ulcerations in the digestive tract, where they take up residence. In severe cases their activity can create anemia as a result of blood loss. Blackish stool is a telltale sign. Cats may become infected from maternal milk that contains worms or by eating affected rodents. Hookworms are more of a kitten problem. Mature cats may be affected if they are exposed to kennels, crowded environments, cat shows, or other stressful situations.

Dewormer Plus Natural Remedies—Joseph Demers, DVM

If hookworms are detected through a stool test, the veterinarian can prescribe the appropriate dewormer medication. Some holistic-minded pet owners may balk at the suggestion of using a chemical dewormer, but it works very well to quickly eliminate a worm over-load. You need to use it only for a day or two. After the treatment, you can start rebuilding the animal's health with a comprehensive supplement program. Included among my recommendations are digestive enzymes and probiotics. Probiotic supplements restore beneficial bacteria to the gastrointestinal tract that are destroyed by antibiotics, dewormers, and other medications. I use a combined enzyme and probiotic formula called FloraZyme LP, made by Pet's Friends, Inc. (954-720-0794). It can be used short-term after deworming or on a long-term basis for general health.

PRODUCTS AND DOSAGE

- **Pet digestive enzyme.** They aid the digestive system. Follow label instructions. Give for two to three months.

- **Probiotic supplement.** This restores beneficial microorganisms that have been destroyed in the gut by the dewormer. Give for two weeks.

- **Hematinic.** This is a blood-building nutritional supplement with B-complex vitamins and iron. Available in pet stores. Follow label instructions. Use for one month.

- **Tang Kwei Gin,** a Chinese herbal blood-building preparation that helps to boost the immune system and recovery of an animal. Available in Chinese pharmacies or groceries, where it may also be known as Imperial Tang Kwei Gin. The formula is prepared as a liquid remedy in single-dose vials, similar to how ginseng is often packaged. Give 1/4 vial to a kitten twice daily for ten days.

Wormwood Vs. Hookworm—Karen Bentley, DVM

Wormwood Combination, developed by herbalist Hanna Kroeger, is beneficial for mild cases of hookworm. The formula contains black walnut leaves, wormwood, quassia, cloves, and male fern. The product is available through Hanna's Herb Shop, in Boulder, Colorado, at 800-206-6722.

Hookworms should always be first treated chemically. The herbal combo can then be used daily for two weeks to help prevent reinfestation. It is quite useful alone in this capacity for animals constantly reinfecting themselves, such as cats who are hunters and catch infected rodents and birds.

DOSAGE

- 1/4 capsule daily for two weeks twice a year (spring and fall). Open capsule and mix in food. Give for two weeks every three months if cat continually reinfects itself.

ROUNDWORMS

Roundworms, cream colored and up to five inches long, are the most common intestinal parasite of cats. They are estimated to affect between one-quarter and three-quarters of adult cats. The most common source of infection is ingestion of infected mice, birds, or insects. Among kittens the incidence may be even higher, a result of the parasites being passed through the mother's milk. Regardless of the cleanliness in the household or breeding facility, this parasite is extremely effective in transporting itself from one generation to the next.

Unlike other worms, you won't see the typical signs such as worms being passed out in the stool. The most common sign of roundworm infestation in cats is a ravenous appetite. The big appetite could also be a thyroid condition, so it is important to get a veterinarian's opinion whenever you notice a change in the animal's usual habits.

Roundworms are not considered as "lethal" as other parasites; nevertheless if left untreated, they can cause inflammation and blockage in the gut, the absorption of toxins into the body, and, if enough of them have migrated out of the intestines, damage to organs such as the liver and lungs. Infected kittens are in particular risk if not treated.

Chemical Dewormer Plus Enzymes—Ron Carsten, DVM

I have had excellent results with Zymex II, made by Standard Process (800-848-5061; sold through veterinarians). This supplement, containing digestive enzymes, literally consumes parasites present in the upper-intestinal tract. It can be given by itself, but it takes about six weeks to work and is much more expensive than many of the new safe and effective chemical dewormers. I typically use a chemical dewormer to get rid of the worms quickly and then recommend Zymex II preventively once a week. This approach works well as a general strategy, particularly if you live in an area with a known roundworm problem or if your animal is constantly exposed to roundworms.

DOSAGE
- **Zymex II:** 1 capsule daily on an empty stomach.

Wormwood for Roundworms—Karen Bentley, DVM

I recommend Hanna Kroeger's Wormwood Combination (see Bentley's entry under hookworms).

DOSAGE
- 1/4 capsule daily. Combination can be used for two weeks at a time twice yearly, or even four times, if necessary, for cats who become constantly reinfected.

SCREW WORMS (MAGGOTS)

Clear Skin Wounds with Charcoal—Roger DeHaan, DVM

Maggots that develop at the site of an injury or wound can burrow into the skin, devour flesh, and create infections. You can effectively get rid of them by using wood ash or charcoal. First clean out the wound with a Q-tip soaked with hydrogen peroxide. Then apply the charcoal or ash. Do this twice a day. The charcoal or ash is very alkaline and will kill the maggots.

TAPEWORMS

Cats typically develop tapeworms by swallowing fleas during grooming that have in turn eaten tapeworm eggs, or by eating infected rodents. You may notice ricelike particles in the stool or sticking to the anal hair. These may be tapeworm segments. Tapeworms are large parasites that live in the gut. They often migrate to the anus, which leads to irritating itching. Often an infected cat will drag its rear end on the ground because of the itching. In large numbers, tapeworms can cause weight loss, diarrhea, and debility. While the sight of tapeworm segments may be alarming, these parasites are seldom the cause of severe illness.

Granatum (Homeopathic)—Charles Loops, DVM

The homeopathic remedy Granatum works effectively to rid animals who have occasional tapeworm problems. I find it works as well as Dronsit or Cestex, the standard chemical products.

DOSAGE
- **Granatum 6X or 12X,** four times a day for five days. It may be difficult to give that many doses a day, but in my experience it requires that much. In some cases you may have to repeat the process the following week. If an animal has a continual tapeworm problem, it will require an individualized homeopathic program beyond just giving Granatum.

Homeopathic Combination—Stan Gorlitsky, DVM

For more than ten years I have use a homeopathic mother tincture combination of Gnaphalium and Filix mas that is highly effective in ridding animals of chronic tapeworm problems. The remedy, called Tape Away, is available through my clinic at 803-881-9915. It has no side effects. Generally I recommend first using one of the standard tapeworm medications to clean out the animal and then following with the remedy on a regular basis for prevention. However, the remedy can be effective without the medication. Worms are usually eliminated within a week.

DOSAGE
- If used in connection with a conventional dewormer, give a few drops for two or three days twice a month after having completed treatment with the medication. If used by itself, give a few drops twice daily for a week to ten days on a monthly basis.

Prevent Tapeworm with Herbs—Karen Bentley, DVM
To help prevent tapeworms, I recommend Hanna Kroeger's Rascal herbal worming formula, containing pumpkin seed, garlic, crampbark, capsicum, and thyme.

DOSAGE
- 1/4 capsule daily for two weeks twice a year (spring and fall). Open capsule and mix in food. If animal has a chronic flea problem and constantly reinfects itself, use the preparation daily for two weeks every three months.

⚹ Poisoning, ⚹ Drug Side Effects, and Toxicity

For acute cases of poisoning, see a veterinarian immediately; for gastrointestinal upsets related to antibiotic use, see "Diarrhea" in Digestive Disorders

POISONING

Activated Charcoal for Poisoning—Roger DeHaan, DVM
For emergency situations over weekends or where you can't get to a veterinarian, activated charcoal is a great remedy. This is for the quick response, where your animal has gotten into a bottle of medicine, raided the neighbor's garbage can, or eaten a poisonous plant or rotting fish on the beach. You can purchase it at health food stores or through Holistic Veterinary Services (218-846-9112).

Activated charcoal is a time-tested, primary remedy that is always safe and never contraindicated. You almost can't give too much of it in situations like these.

The secret of activated charcoal is its adsorption power—that is, its ability to draw poison to itself, form a permanent bond with the poison, and escort it out of the body. Charcoal is the black part of partially burned wood. In folk medicine it has long been used as a remedy for many poisons and is referred to as "the universal antidote."

Activated charcoal means the wood has gone through a special process of slow burning in a pit under oxygen deprivation, which gives it several times the "binding power" of normal charcoal. The substance can hold many times its own weight in toxic substances.

If an animal ingests a toxic substance and vomiting immediately occurs, then there is really no crisis. The concern is if the poison is not vomited from the system. The charcoal benefits the animal by adsorbing whatever poison is present in the system and eliminating it through the bowel. But in any case, see your veterinarian or nearest emergency clinic as soon as possible.

Charcoal can be given as a capsule, but also opened and syringed or force fed in any food the pet likes, such as yogurt, apple sauce or chicken broth. The powder is black and messy, but can make a difference in a time of crisis.

The U.S. Food and Drug Administration rates activated charcoal as effective in adsorbing many drugs, poisons, and gases. Today you will find this substance in most hospital emergency rooms, where it is used for drug overdoses and accidental poisonings.

DOSAGE
- Give 2 capsules, or 1 teaspoon of powder (mixed in liquid) depending on potential severity of poisoning. Then call your veterinarian. Treatment may be repeated in ten to thirty minutes.

POISONING FROM MEDICATIONS

According to the American Veterinary Medical Association, drugs are by far the most common type of small-animal poison exposure. Human over-the-counter pain relievers are occasionally used in veterinary medicine but should be given only if a veterinarian specifically directs you to do so. While safe for us, these products are not designed for pets, and a minimal human dose can poison an animal. As little as 1 regular-strength tablet (325 milligrams) of acetaminophen (Tylenol), for instance, can cause noticeable signs of illness. Two extra-strength tablets can kill a cat. Felines are also sensitive to aspirin.

For an excellent overview of common poison dangers, refer to the American Veterinary Medical Association's "Pet Poison Guide" on the organization's Web site. The Internet address is http:www.avma.org/pubhlth/poisgde.html.

Beware of Willow Bark—Nancy Scanlan, DVM

The herb willow bark is often used for pain. But be aware that it has the potential to cause more ulcers than buffered aspirin. Anything in the aspirin family, including willow bark, can be particularly toxic for cats. I don't recommend its use for cats.

TOXICITY

As horrible as it sounds, many of us are toxic waste dumps, our inner machinery clogged with environmental chemicals, pharmaceutical drugs, and contaminants from the environment. Unfortunately most people are unaware that accumulated toxicity in the body is a common underlying cause for many conditions and symptoms of fatigue, pain, and general unwellness. Unless we rid the body of these poisons, they continue to build up and erode health and vitality. Marshall Mandell, M.D., an expert in environmental medicine, puts it this way: "Everything that we eat, drink, or inhale is now polluted with chemical agents that are foreign to our bodily chemistry, and we are suffering the consequences of possessing a body that is incapable of handling the by-products of our own amazing chemical technology."

The same holds true for cats.

"I see this in my practice all the time," says Mark Haverkos, DVM, of Oldenburg, Indiana. "The sick animals I see are very toxic, a result of the toxic food and medicine they take and the less-than-pure air and water."

Holistic veterinarians routinely consider the problem of toxicity in their treatment strategies. Here are some suggestions they offer for measures you can take on your own to reduce the toxic level in your animals.

Homeopathic Detox Par Excellence—Mark Haverkos, DVM

Increasingly, I have to detoxify animals as a first step in the healing process. A big tip for keeping animals healthy or when starting them on the road to recovery is to do a periodic detoxification. That's a great place to start any kind of an alternative program. All you need is a bottle of the homeopathic remedy Nux vomica, available at any health food store.

In more than half the cases I see, a round of Nux vomica lessens the severity of the symptoms, whatever they are. A woman brought in a two-year-old domestic shorthair who had been urinating outside the litter box. She thought it was straining. Another veterinarian had given the cat an antibiotic that didn't help. I put the cat on a one-week course of Nux vomica 30C. Within four days the symptoms were gone.

Another cat was presented with a discharge from the eyes. Previously the cat had been treated with ophthalmic ointment and antibiotics. I gave the cat owner some eyedrops and Nux vomica and the situation quickly resolved.

Animals have more energy, interest in their surroundings, and just plain more wellness when they are cleaned out. Nux is good for most cases except when an animal is very weak or near death.

Unless an animal has been raised totally organic, never been vaccinated, fed only clean food since early in life, and provided a lot of fresh air and exercise, I almost automatically reach for the Nux vomica whenever the animal comes in the door.

DOSAGE
- **Nux vomica (6C to 30C potencies)** once a day until you start to see changes, and then stop the remedy.

Herb and Flower Combo Detoxifier—Shannon Hines, DVM

For a general detoxification of the system, I use Detoxifier for Cats, a liquid formula combining herbs and flower essences made by Tasha's Herbs (800-315-0142). It helps clean out animals who have been on long-term medication or who are exposed to constant low-grade toxicity in the environment, such as from lawn chemicals. The formula includes cornsilk, burdock root, Siberian ginseng, licorice root, milk thistle seed, yellow dock, and dandelion root. The product includes cod liver oil, vitamin E, and lecithin for extra nutrition and to accommodate feline tastes.

DOSAGE
• Follow label instructions.

Better Nutrition Equals Fewer Side Effects—Roger DeHaan, DVM

All pharmaceutical drugs are toxic to the body. And all create side effects to some degree. Some animals do fine on prescription drugs. Others do not. Over the years I have learned that animals with good nutritional status are better equipped to counteract drug toxicity. If they are poorly nourished, they generally have less ability to detoxify drugs. Good nutrition is vital, whether animals are on drugs or herbs. The more malnourished they are, the more likely they are to have reactions.

Milk Thistle Detox—Pamela Wood-Krzeminski, DVM

The herb milk thistle (*Silymarin*) is a magnificent protector and detoxifier of the liver. It is used to treat acute liver toxicity in people. I use the Twin Labs silymarin extract, available in health food stores.

For cats, I recommend milk thistle for any animal who has been on any kind of medication, or who is being maintained on long-term medication, or who has undergone surgical or dental procedures involving the use of anesthesia.

I consider milk thistle a *must*, for instance, for any epileptic animal maintained on anticonvulsive drugs. I would have the animal stay on the milk thistle for as long as it is on the drug. There is no known contraindication or interference with medications.

Milk thistle specifically helps heal liver cells damaged from medication or anesthesia. In the case of short-term medication, milk thistle may not be necessary, but it can't hurt.

DOSAGE
- 1 capsule daily. You can empty the contents in water or mix with the animal's regular food or a meaty baby food.

⤹ Pregnancy, Nursing, and Beyond ⤸

If ever there was a time to improve the nutrition of an animal, this is it. Holistic veterinarians encourage clients to provide the best possible diet to pregnant and lactating females and to supplement the diet with at least a high-quality multi-vitamin-mineral formula for pets. Pregnancy and lactation cause severe biochemical stress. The bitch is providing for anywhere from two to half a dozen or more kittens. She must herself be nutritionally fit if she is to pass on the necessary nutrients to her progeny.

FLOWER ESSENCES
(See chapter 10 for general guidelines on flower essences.)

Rescue Remedy for Weak Kittens—A. Greig Howie, DVM
Rescue Remedy, the popular flower essence, benefits weak kittens and helps them cope with stress, shock, and trauma.

DOSAGE
- Dilute it according to the label directions and then administer a couple of drops in the mouth. You can give it every few minutes as needed until the animal perks up.

HERBS

Raspberry Leaves for Easier Birthing—Lynne Friday, DVM

Raspberry leaf tea helps accelerate and ease the birthing process. I recommend it for any pregnant animal. It is available in health food stores.

Start giving it a month before breeding and throughout the pregnancy. To help clean out the insides, give it for several weeks afterward.

This simple step consistently helps animals, but don't expect it to work with Persians and Himalayans and any distorted-face breed. You can give them tea until raspberries grow out of their ears, but those birth canals were just not meant to accommodate the unnatural faces that these poor animals have been bred for.

Dosage
- Put 1 teabag in 1 quart of boiling water. Let steep until the color resembles maple syrup. Cover well and store it in the refrigerator. Dole out the quart during one week. Pour onto the animal's food.

Chamomile Eases Teething—Jan Bellows, DVM

For the discomfort of teething, chamomile works very well to decrease swelling and soothe the disturbed gum tissue. A sign of discomfort is an animal pawing at its mouth.

Boil a teabag, then put the bag in the refrigerator and apply it cold to the gums. Do this two or three times a day for a few moments at a time until the teeth come in.

HOMEOPATHIC REMEDIES

Phytolacca for Mastitis—A. Greig Howie, DVM

Phytolacca 30C alleviates about 75 percent of mastitis cases. The condition is characterized by redness and swelling, usually of one particular gland, and the mother will not want any of the little ones to nurse from that gland. You can also apply hot packs to the area to help resolve the problem. If the animal goes off food or develops a fever, be sure to see a veterinarian at once.

DOSAGE
- A few drops in the mouth three times a day until the condition improves.

NUTRITIONAL SUPPLEMENTS

Vitamin C for Kittenhood and Beyond—Nino Aloro, DVM
Kittens benefit from extra vitamin C. The vitamin enhances the immune system and contributes to healthier tissue, including strong teeth.

DOSAGE
- Start with 50 milligrams twice daily and increase slowly to 250 milligrams twice daily. Adult cats can be maintained at that level. Increase to 1,000 milligrams if the animal becomes ill.

FOOD AND SPECIAL DIETS

Too Much Kitty Food—William Pollak, DVM
The leading problem among kittens is man-made: poor quality and excess quantity of food. So many people overfeed their young animals, which frequently results in diarrhea. The animals simply don't have enough enzymes to break down the quantity of food they are given. They are also getting too much grain to eat (see Pollak's recommendation for feeding in chapter 6).

Improve the Diet—Norman C. Ralston, DVM
There is no substitute for anything less than the best possible nutrition. If your pregnant cat is eating a commercial food diet, slowly add some good natural and unprocessed ingredients. Examples would be a teaspoonful of grated raw or lightly steams carrots, chopped leafy greens, cabbage, or squash. Then add up to 25 percent raw or lightly cooked fish, preferably the white fish variety.

INTRODUCING SOLIDS TO KITTENS
A good way to introduce solid food to a kitten is to take a small piece of raw ground beef, about the size of a small bean. Flatten it between the forefinger and the thumb and then dip it into an egg yolk previously separated from the white. This egg yolk–dipped beef bit is

then placed in the mouth of each kitten. It is amazing how this seems to stimulate their appetite for solid food.

FINDING AND CARING FOR KITTENS

Match the Cat to the Home—Paul McCutcheon, DVM

- Try to match an animal's temperament to the environment you have in mind for it. Choose your animal well. Once you choose, try to keep down the stress level. Kittenhood is an extremely stressful time for an animal. Not only are there dramatic changes, separation from mother and litter, but there is also a rapid growth cycle. Seek out the advice of a behaviorist who can help you train and integrate the animal into the projected surroundings. Poor training results in added stress for the animal—and you. Added stress increases the risk of illness and makes for an unhappy animal. If your animal will be alone much of the time, you need to train it that way. Look ahead.

- Introduce your new kitten to the litter box immediately and make sure it is easily accessible at all times. Kittens will instinctively use the box. However, if you notice the cat squatting elsewhere, place the animal into the box. Clean the box daily.

Choose a Healthy Cat and Keep It Healthy—Jean Hofve, DVM

- When you pick a kitten, look for an animal that radiates health. Check for eye discharges. Look in the ears. If you see what looks like coffee grinds in there, that means ear mites. Check the litter box for signs of diarrhea. Look at the belly. A swollen belly full of air could indicate the presence of worms.

- It is not necessary to feed a kitten diet. People use these far too long. Foods formulated for all life stages are fine.

- Get kittens started on meat. Kittens will eat any kind of meat anytime. They have not had their taste buds wrecked by years of commercial cat food. Use a variety of meats. If you feed a commercial diet, be sure to supplement animals with meat.

- Feed frequently. Feed all they want. Kittens don't get fat as a rule.

- Train kittens early to use a scratching post. It is extremely difficult, if not impossible, to train an adult cat to do that. Use a post at least three feet high, or it won't be tall enough when the cat is full-grown.

- When you play with a kitten, don't use your bare hands or allow it to bite or scratch bare skin. Use rolled-up socks or toys. If a kitty starts gnawing on your hand, relax your hand. The kitten will lose interest in anything that isn't moving. Don't try to pull away. You may get hurt when it clamps down to try to keep the hand there. It may be fun and appear harmless when they are small, but adult cats in the habit of biting are dangerous. Don't let them develop the habit.

- If you don't want the cat to be an outdoor animal, don't let it out—ever, not in the yard and not on a leash. Once you do, you have created a cat who knows now that looking out the window is not watching "kitty TV" but that there is a real world out there, and it will want to be a part of it.

☙ Skin Disorders and Allergies ❧

See also Fleas, Ticks, and Insect Pests; Food Allergies

The disturbing sight of a cat constantly scratching or chewing on its skin drives pet owners to veterinary clinics en masse for help. Skin disorders are, in fact, the number one problem treated by veterinarians.

The causes are many, and often in combination. Among the major offenders:

- Flea-bite sensitivities, the most common cause of skin problems (see section on fleas).
- Poor nutrition.
- Food allergies (see section on food allergies).

- Dust, mold, and chemical sensitivities.
- Reactions to vaccinations (see chapter 14).
- Stress (see following section on stress).
- Excessive licking from boredom.

The most common allergy-related skin condition is known as "miliary dermatitis," a term going back to earlier days when people described their cats as having grains of millet under the skin. You will see small bumps, sores, and scabs usually in the area of the head, neck, and back.

So-called rodent ulcers occur generally in female cats and involve a thickening, reddish inflammation of the lips, lesions on the tummy, and rashes that develop on the backside of the rear legs.

A problem called "eosinophilic plaques" causes intense licking and scratching of raised sores on the abdomen or inside thigh.

Another common condition is feline acne. You will see a blackhead or zitlike outbreak on the chin. The pimples are often full of a bloody pus, indicative of a bacterial infection.

Finding an effective treatment for these and other feline skin disorders is often quite challenging. Veterinarians usually resort to steroids, antibiotics, antihistamines, and sometimes even tranquilizers. These approaches may temporarily stop scratching, but if used over a long period of time, they can negatively affect the adrenal glands, liver, and kidneys. Holistic veterinarians criticize the reliance on drugs for symptoms of chronic skin problems.

The skin is the body's largest organ of detoxification, and a rash or irritation is a natural way of eliminating a toxin. "Hot spots," for instance, may develop as a result of the body trying to rid itself of toxins or of inner heat generated by poor-quality dry food being constantly fed to an animal.

"When the condition is treated with drugs, the activity of the immune system is suppressed, and the toxin is prevented from leaving the body," says Robert Goldstein, VMD. "Sometimes giving drugs is appropriate, but reliance on drugs alone over the long term is asking for a chronic, never-ending skin condition as well as other health problems."

Drug treatments may help for a while, but months later animals are frequently back in the clinic with renewed symptoms and some-times new problems, involving perhaps the kidneys or wherever there is a genetic weakness. Such new problems may appear unre-lated but in reality may be part of an unaddressed continuum of the same imbalances or disease processes still raging inside the animal.

Properly used steroids can relieve inflammation and control itch-ing, but they are often misused and overdosed. Problems frequently occur when animals are put on arbitrary levels that are beyond what they need.

WHY SKIN ALLERGIES?

"A common saying is that if your pet is a face rubber, foot licker, and armpit scratcher, then he's probably allergic to something," says Ernest K. Smith, DVM, secretary of the Academy of Veterinary Allergy and Clinical Immunology, as quoted in a 1994 article in the *Orange County* (California) *Register.*

Medical dictionaries define an allergy as "a hypersensitive state acquired through exposure to a particular allergen." An allergen is any substance that can cause an immediate or delayed reaction. For pets it is most commonly a protein in the saliva of fleas that bite the animal. But it can also be other insect bites, as well as pollen, dust, mold, food, chemicals, and wool.

Humans sniffle, sneeze, cough, and wheeze when their bodies have been "insulted" by an allergen. But cats most frequently itch and develop skin disorders, although felines with inhalant allergies can develop asthma where they, too, cough, wheeze, and experience difficulty in breathing.

The difference has to do with mast cells, specialized cells in the body that respond to allergens by production of a chemical called histamine. It is the release of histamine that triggers symptoms by causing small blood vessels to leak and ooze fluid, resulting in a swelling of tissue. In humans the mast cells are highly concentrated in the area of the eyes, nose, and windpipe. That's why people with hay fever experience nasal congestion, a result of leaky vessels and swelling in the nose. In animals the cells are concentrated on the sides of the face, paws, armpit, and groin. That's why animals rub, scratch, chew, or lick in those areas.

Many sensitive people are intolerant to multiple substances. This can cause unique combinations of physical, mental, emotional, and behavioral symptoms. The same is true for animals. Skin is affected most frequently, but intestinal disorders, behavioral disturbances, seizures, and other problems also occur, both with or without a concurrent skin problem. New allergies can arise any time an animal is exposed to any substance for a period of time. Some allergic reactions appear after exposure to a single allergen. Others appear only after exposure to multiple substances. It depends on an animal's individual resistance.

A GROWING PROBLEM IN YOUNGER ANIMALS

In 1986 Los Angeles veterinarian Alfred Plechner, DVM, and I collaborated on a book about pet allergies *(Pet Allergies: Remedies for an Epidemic)*. It was Plechner's opinion, based on years of clinical experience, that an unrecognized allergy epidemic was ruining the health of millions of pets. The situation hasn't changed and if anything has only gotten worse, he says today.

Plechner continually sees cats with inferior or damaged immunity, who are seriously affected by environmental input. "This is a major problem," he says. "Perhaps one out of two animals brought in to veterinary hospitals may be suffering from some degree of allergic malady, a hypersensitive state that can cause death and not just everyday scratching problems. Allergies are so common that pet owners probably face the problem sometime or another during the life of their animals."

Adds Joseph Demers, DVM: "I now see many more allergies than before—the result, I believe, of a confused or out-of-balance immune system underreacting or overreacting, or otherwise just not doing its normal job. Years ago I used to see this in animals two or more years of age, and now I see allergies in animals as young as six months of age. Cats under a year of age are coming in with severe skin allergies."

The main reasons for this situation are these:

- **Flawed food.** Commercial pet foods are loaded with highly processed, inferior-quality ingredients and chemicals that may contribute to overall ill health or trigger allergic sensitivities. Feeding the same food continually could set off an allergic reaction that manifests as itchy skin.

- **Cosmetic breeding.** Many cats have entered the world burdened with genetic weaknesses due to selective breeding practices, where animals are bred for certain features valued by fanciers and cat show judges. This translates into prestige and maximum sales prices for breeders, whose standards are then mass-produced by kitty mills. The result is wholesale merchandising of fashionable animals who have distorted hormonal and immune function, less coping ability, and health problems showing up at ever younger ages. Such biological weaknesses are passed on to purebred offspring and to mixed-breed descendants as well.

- **Overvaccinating.** The current use of powerful and multiple vaccines creates a "massive insult to the immune system," leading to general dysfunction and allergies, says Demers. Skin problems frequently develop within a few months of vaccination. Holistic veterinarians are very aware of this generally overlooked connection. Vaccination will probably aggravate your animal's skin if it already has an allergic skin condition (itchiness and rashes) or has ever been treated with steroids for a skin condition. If you have any questions about vaccinating, ask your veterinarian. Don't vaccinate unnecessarily. Homeopathic remedies are highly effective in preventing and clearing up reactions (see chapter 14 on vaccinations and how to prevent and treat reactions).

- **Proliferation of chemicals.** This is an age of unprecedented proliferation of chemicals and pollutants that many experts say is weakening our immune systems and undermining health. Doris Rapp, M.D., an expert on environmental medicine, says that "if this had happened over hundreds of years, perhaps we could have adapted. Unless our nutrition is good, we can't hope to detoxify these things. But our nutrition has deteriorated over the last half century as well. The food is processed, pesticided, and poor in nutrients. What we drink is full of chemicals. The result is that our bodies have become toxic dump sites." The same situation applies to our companion animals. Cats, with their noses close to the ground and carpets, are intimately exposed to a multitude of toxins: lawn and garden chemicals, rat poison, pesticides, cleaning and disinfectant chemicals, lead in paint and water, building and decorating chemicals, and the fumes outgassing from synthetic carpets. The food they eat is full of chemical additives.

WHY DOES AN ANIMAL DEVELOP SYMPTOMS AT A CERTAIN TIME?

Problems can develop at any time in an animal's life. Imagine your body, or your animal's body, as a barrel that can hold a specific amount of stress and toxins. Each barrel has a different capacity—or threshold—depending on individual genetic strengths or weaknesses. Lifestyle, diet, environmental factors, and chemical exposures are common elements in our lives that cause the barrel to overflow or not. When the barrel overflows, symptoms appear.

If, for instance, you are exposed to a small amount of dust and mold, your barrel—if it is normal—should have the capacity to hold it. But if on another occasion you are exposed to too much of any one or more pollutants, your barrel may overflow. You develop symptoms. Another person in the same circumstances may develop symptoms earlier or later, depending on the size of his or her barrel. If there is much stress in your life at one particular point, or if the weather is very hot, or you are constantly exposed to a certain chemical, your barrel may fill up and overflow faster.

For animals, the combination of poor food, vaccinations, and the advent of flea season offers an obvious seasonal explanation for the barrel spilling over. For many animals, the barrel may always be close to overflowing because of genetic weakness. In such cases it doesn't take much for symptoms to appear. A genetically weak animal on a poor diet and exposed to stress and multiple chemicals is a prime candidate for allergies and illnesses early on.

HOW TO TELL IF YOUR CAT IS ALLERGIC

The following symptoms are typical signs, but not necessarily the only ones, indicating an allergic problem:

- Persistent biting, licking, or scratching of skin.
- Inflamed skin, lumps, bumps, or sores that recur
- Inflamed ears with repeated infections.

GENERAL TIPS TO CONTROL SKIN DISORDERS AND ALLERGIES

There are often no simple answers to allergies. But the following tips will help:

- Feed a better diet. Supplement the diet with vitamins and minerals. This should boost resistance so that fewer drugs may be needed for control. With luck you may even be able to eliminate medication altogether. Whatever the level of your animal's resistance, you have the power to improve it and lessen the potential or intensity of skin allergies.

- Switch to higher-quality protein foods. Better-quality protein has fewer potential allergenic offenders. Changing to a more natural or wholesome diet may reduce allergic reactions. Raw meat fed to cats has been found to reduce allergy problems.

- "Usually there is a combination of things relating to allergic conditions, such as pollen, food, and fleas," says A. Greig Howie, DVM. "If you can eliminate just one of the things, you may be able to bring the allergy back down below the problem threshold."

- Antibiotics can contribute to allergies by destroying the beneficial natural bacteria in the gut. This allows pathogenic organisms to flourish and often creates gastrointestinal upsets that develop into secondary skin disorders. If your animal is on a course of prescribed antibiotics, give it a half capsule of *Lactobacillus acidophilus* per meal. Acidophilus is available in health food stores. It is a strain of important, beneficial bacteria.

- Animals are exposed to many toxic chemicals that may cause reactions. If possible, use natural, nontoxic products in your house and yard.

- Keep down dust levels inside the house. Consider filtration systems.

- Frequent shampooing can provide temporary relief by getting offending "stuff" off the hair coat. If a shampoo is going to help, it should give relief for twelve to forty-eight hours. If not, try another shampoo.

- If you have an allergic animal, consider switching from plastic to ceramic feeding bowls. "I have seen cases where plastic bowls have caused local allergic reactions around the face," says Carvel Tiekert, DVM. "Red bowls seem to evoke more reaction than other colors, but we don't know why."

HERBS

Chinese Herbs for Itchy Skin—Stan Gorlitsky, DVM

For any kind of itchy skin problem, I developed a Chinese herbal combination called Skineze, available through Good Communications at 800-968-1738. The product contains angelica root, the fruit of the burdock plant, calamus gum, Chinese foxglove root, and licorice root. It comes as a chewable tablet with liver flavoring and whey added to make it palatable. The tablets can be crumbled and mixed into food or given intact. Skineze can be used in conjunction with any medication prescribed by a veterinarian.

The formula has a powerful effect. More than two thousand animals have used the product to date, and I estimate that it has significantly helped up to 75 percent of them. It reduces itching that may be due to food allergies and flea or other insect bites. It does not cure the cause of the itching, but it usually provides relief and comfort.

Many cats experience relief within four to twenty-four hours, but some have taken up to a month, particularly in cases involving major hot spots. In about 12 percent of cases the formula has had no effect. In a handful of animals there were minor gastrointestinal side effects that cleared up when the formula was stopped or given in smaller amounts.

Because the product contains whey (for sweetness), don't give it to an animal allergic to dairy. More scratching may result. For such cases we have the same product available in capsule form without any flavoring. The taste is bitter, but sensitive animals usually respond well.

DOSAGE
- Follow label instructions.

Topical Relief with Ayurvedic Gel—Jody Kincaid, DVM

For dealing on the outside with a wide variety of skin problems, including minor injuries, infections, eczema, and hot spots, I have been impressed by Phytogel, an Ayurvedic herbal gel from India that significantly enhances healing. The product is available from Ayuvet (888-881-8767). A small amount goes a long way. It has a pleasant cedar smell that comes from the Himalayan cedarwood oil used in the formulation. Research has shown that cedarwood has antibacterial and antifungal activity. The product also contains neem seed oil, a phytochemical known for its antibacterial and healing properties.

Phytogel has a first-class disinfectant and soothing action and reduces itching and irritation. It works as well as any cortisone cream I have used. One of its features is that once you put on the gel, it will usually stay on. The herbal taste is a deterrent to licking off the gel.

DOSAGE
- Follow label instructions.

Relief with Ayurvedic Herbs Orally—Tejinder Sodhi, DVM

To help skin problems from the inside out, I recommend an Ayurvedic herbal combination called Neem Plus, available from Ayush Herbs (800-925-1371). The product is available in liquid form for cats. It features neem, a well-known Indian herb with a long healing tradition for skin conditions. Research has demonstrated neem's antifungal, antibacterial, and antiviral properties. The product also contains amla, bahera, and haritaki, the three fruit components of triphala, the traditional Indian herbal preparation used as an intestinal cleanser. Triphala adds effectiveness to the formula because many skin conditions are related to intestinal disorders.

Neem Plus is also helpful in cases of yeast infections that many animals develop as an aftermath of antibiotic treatments.

DOSAGE
- 10 drops per ten pounds of body weight twice daily.

HOMEOPATHIC REMEDIES
(See chapter 9 for general dosage guidelines.)

Cooling "Hot Spots" with Arnica—Thomas Van Cise, DVM
"Hot spots," also known as "wet eczema," refers to the all-too-common condition of open sores that are constantly being bitten, scratched, or chewed by animals. Arnica is a good homeopathic remedy to defuse the intensity of itching. The remedy seems to "put out the fire" in the skin.

DOSAGE
- **Arnica 30C:** Give twice daily for two or three days. Observe the results. Don't repeat the remedy as long as you see signs of improvement. If the problem persists, give again for two to three days. Follow this approach as long as you have the problem.

SULFUR FOR SMELLY OR SWEATY SKIN
If you are dealing with a chronic seborrheal-like odor that is not the usual cat smell, use the homeopathic remedy Sulfur.

DOSAGE
- **Sulfur 30C:** Give once a day for two or three days.

NUTRITIONAL SUPPLEMENTS

B Complex Plus Amino Acids—Nino Aloro, DVM
For years I have successfully used a combination of B-complex vitamins and a multiple amino acid formula to improve the health of the

skin and support any medical treatment. The B-complex product is called Lipocaps, made by Vetus Animal Health and distributed by Burns Veterinary Supply (800-922-8767). The amino multi is Pure Form Amino Acids, from Jo-Mar Labs (800-538-4545).

Some clients have told me that skin problems return whenever they run out of the supplements.

DOSAGE
- **Lipocaps:** 1 capsule daily.

- **Pure Form Amino Acids:** 1 or 2 capsules daily.

Vitamin C, Pantothenic Acid, Fatty Acids—Carvel Tiekert, DVM

Vitamin C, pantothenic acid (a B-complex vitamin), and fatty acids offer a simple, inexpensive, and helpful approach. C and pantothenic acid can have a significant effect. They are important immune boosters with the potential to increase resistance to allergens. Allergic response is basically the result of a dysfunctional immune system. Vitamin C and pantothenic acid alone generate good results fairly quickly in about 30 percent of cases. If you don't see improvement in a week, this approach is not going to have any major benefits. If response is good, reduce the dose and frequency to the lowest effective level. Vitamin C can be given in any form, although I like nonacidic sodium or calcium ascorbate in the powder form.

Omega-3 fatty acids are well documented in veterinary research literature to help against skin-related allergies by promoting the production of natural anti-inflammatory substances in the body. I use Opticoat II, made by Natural Animal Nutrition (800-548-2899), as my fatty acid supplement. It contains flaxseed oil, marine lipids, and vitamin E and alone will control allergic dermatitis in 10 percent of cases. About half of the time this product allows me to cut back on other therapies.

DOSAGE
- **Vitamin C:** 500 milligrams daily

- **Pantothenic acid:** 100 milligrams twice a day.

- **Opticoat II:** Follow label instructions.

Enzymes Plus Trace Minerals—Alfred Plechner, DVM

For combating skin problems, a plant-based digestive enzyme supplement for pets is very beneficial. Add it directly into the food. The enzymes improve nutritional absorption. Older or sickly cats are very often deficient in digestive enzymes. Supplementation benefits the entire system, including the skin.

I also recommend a good nutritional supplement with trace minerals because the soil we grow our food in is often deficient in minerals. Minerals are the building materials of strong bones, tissue, teeth, nails, and hair coat. Along with the major minerals, such as calcium, magnesium, potassium, and zinc, there are dozens of other lesser-known elements—needed in tiny, trace amounts—that are important for health. Mineral deficiencies are involved in many common disorders. I reached this conclusion through the simple step of supplementing the diets of animals with natural products containing seventy or so different minerals. Supplementation with minerals is highly beneficial. Within a six-month period I usually see the following results:

- Improvement in general health.
- Darker, thicker hair coat with increased luster.
- Reduced scratching.
- Reduced flakiness.
- Better maintenance of body weight with reduced caloric intake.
- In geriatric cats, increased activity and improved condition of hair coat.
- Animals plagued by fleas appear to be less attractive to insects. You can see that effect usually within a few weeks.

Many of my clients supplement enzymes and trace minerals for both healing and general prevention. I recommend a palatable product called Power for Life, made by Terra Oceana (805-563-2634), which contains an effective array of enzymes, nutrients, and trace minerals. When dealing with a skin problem, use the enzymes and minerals therapeutically for seven days straight and check for progress. If you don't see improvement by that time, continue the supplements but slowly switch your animal to a simple diet of lamb or chicken or any of the hypoallergenic Innovative Veterinary Diet products available through veterinarians.

If you start seeing improvement, start adding back individual foods, a single food a week at a time (see Plechner's add-back plan in the food allergies section). If that approach doesn't work, you probably need to look at imbalances in the animal's hormonal system (see chapter 15 on what to do when nothing works).

Over the years dry, itchy, scaly skin has often been treated with fatty acid supplements. Fatty acids can indeed help the quality of the skin and hair coat if there is a deficiency, which is, in fact, fairly common. However, food allergies, deficiencies in digestive enzymes, and imbalances in hormones can also often create this same unhealthy skin condition. And if there is an enzyme deficiency or imbalance, the fatty acids may not become absorbed and reach the skin. Instead they bind with minerals and fat-soluble vitamins and go out with the stool.

DOSAGE
• **Power for Life:** Follow label instructions.

Fish Oils—Stan Gorlitsky, DVM

If an animal has dry skin with obvious signs of flaky dandruff, I recommend fish oil capsules. You can purchase them in most grocery, drug, or health food stores. Cats love the taste.

DOSAGE
• 1 capsule daily. Prick capsules and squeeze content onto food.

Vitamin C, Antioxidants—Wendell Belfield, DVM

I have developed a simple protocol in my practice, and animals typically show great improvement with it. The total elimination of steroids and other medications is often possible. But it is not a quick fix. The body requires approximately six weeks to adjust to the biochemical changes brought about by this program.

First, feed the best possible diet to your animal. The dry foods I recommend to my clients are made by Natura Pet Products (800-532-7261). For wet food, I suggest Nature's Recipe, available at most pet and food stores.

Add Mega-C Plus, an effective supplement with vitamin C and

extra vitamins and minerals. Supplemental C acts as an antihistamine and also strengthens the immune system. The product is available from Orthomolecular Specialties (408-227-9334).

I also recommend Vital Liquid, an antioxidant combination of vitamins E and A and selenium, also available through Orthomolecular Specialties. This formula protects the body against stress and oxidative damages and helps raise the efficiency of key thyroid and adrenal hormones to boost resistance.

Give both supplements with food.

DOSAGE

- **Mega-C Plus:** Start cats with 750 milligrams of the powder daily, mixed into food. Every third day, increase the dosage by 1/8 teaspoon. When the stool loses its firmness and cylindrical form, decrease one increment level and remain at this daily dosage; this is the bowel tolerance level. At this level the stool should maintain its cylindrical form. Levels will vary from animal to animal. Once the animal is asymptomatic, return to the starting level as a routine maintenance dose.

- **Vital Liquid:** Start cats with 800 IU of vitamin E, 10,000 IU of vitamin A, 20 micrograms of selenium. When symptoms clear up, continue supplementation at a maintenance level as follows: 100 IU of E, 1,250 IU of A, and 2.5 micrograms of selenium.

- **Note:** Animals with immune weakness or imbalances will often regress under stress conditions. In such a case, you need to return immediately to the effective therapeutic levels.

Flaxseed Oil, Vitamin E, and Zinc—Jean Hofve, DVM

This combination works well to relieve and clear up many skin conditions, including miliary dermatitis, feline acne, rodent ulcers, dandruff, and poor hair coat.

Flaxseed oil is excellent for the skin, even though the taste—as far as cats are concerned—leaves much to be desired. Use the sneak attack method, starting with a tiny amount—a few drops—and then increase slowly. I prefer Barlean's organic oil (800-445-3529) for its high quality. The product is readily available in health food stores.

Vitamin E has a long track record for its healing properties and ability to improve skin and coat conditions.

Zinc is good for the skin and particularly for inflammatory conditions. Among other things it speeds the healing of wounds. "Rodent ulcers" often respond well to zinc. I have had some remarkable cures with zinc, but I've also had total failures.

If you don't want to use these three separate ingredients, a good all-in-one substitute is Missing Link, a pet supplement made by Designing Health, Inc. (800-774-7387). The product contains essential fatty acids and many nutritional factors important for healthy skin.

The problem of feline acne can also be helped by using a glass or ceramic feeding bowl instead of a plastic or stainless-steel bowl. Use a bowl that is straight-sided instead of angled. This way the cat is less likely to pick up bacteria or residual food particles on its chin. Keep the bowl very clean.

I recommend giving a cat with acne a daily chin "scrub" or cleansing using Betadine, a liquid antiseptic soap sold in many stores. Add a few drops of the soap in a bowl of warm water to make a *weak* dilution. If you make it too strong, it will irritate the skin. Take a cotton ball, Q-tip, or gauze and apply the solution to the affected areas. Be gentle. Some of the lesions may be painful.

DOSAGE

- **Flaxseed oil:** 1/3 teaspoon daily, or 1–2 eyedroppersful, mixed into the food.

- **Vitamin E:** 200 IU daily.

- **Zinc:** 5 to 10 milligrams for a week or two. If the problem doesn't clear up, discontinue. Zinc can be toxic in overdose.

- **Missing Link:** Follow label instructions.

MIXED AND MISCELLANEOUS APPROACHES

Oxygen for Hot Spots—Thomas Van Cise, DVM

A stabilized oxygen spray product called Earth Bounty Oxy Mist from Matrix Health Products (800-736-5609) works very well for hot spots. This is a human product available in health food stores.

You can spray it on the most purulent drippy sores, the kind where the animal doesn't want you to touch it.

Relief is rapid. Animals often will stop licking or chewing the sore by the end of the first day. Within two to four days you will see substantial healing under way.

For long-haired animals, first trim the long hairs hanging down into the sore. There is no need to do this with short-haired animals.

I previously used calendula topical sprays for this problem and found that they worked better than most commercial veterinary sprays (such as cortisone). But the oxygen spray provides even more rapid and effective relief.

DOSAGE
• Spray sores three times daily.

Healing Oil for Hot Spots—Stan Gorlitsky, DVM

For raw or hot spots, or wounds of any kind, I suggest Healing Oil, a formula I developed with the homeopathic remedies Urtica urens, Symphytum, Calendula, Hypericum, and Arnica in a base of extra-virgin olive oil, plus lavender, chamomile, and geranium oils. The product is available through Good Communications at 800-968-1738. The oil is applied directly to the affected area of the skin. It helps to clean the wound and speed the healing process. I also use it for "dirty" ears and minor ear conditions.

DOSAGE
• Follow label instructions.

Healing from Outside and Inside—Robert Goldstein, VMD

For skin flare-ups and hot spots, I have had good success with a double-barreled inside-outside approach.

OUTSIDE
• First, to soothe skin irritations and help stop the scratching and lick cycle, apply a wet, warm black teabag on the affected spot. This acts in place of a cortisone cream. The tannic acids in the teabag ooze onto the skin and have a soothing itch-relieving effect. Hold the bag to the skin for four or five minutes. Do this twice daily for three days. It is very effective.

- Following the teabag treatments, apply aloe vera gel, either fresh from an opened leaf or from a purchased gel. Aloe speeds the healing process.

INSIDE

Any of the following products can help break the scratch cycle from the inside by strengthening your animal's immune system and increasing the ability to eliminate toxins. Choose one or a combination of these recommendations. When the animal stops scratching, and sore spots on the skin begin to heal and dry over, this is an indication that the itching is gone. At this point the remedies can usually be reduced or discontinued.

- Vitamin B$_6$, a natural antihistamine.

- Either Skin and Seborrhea, by Homeopet (800-423-2256), or Scratch Free, made by Dr. Goodpet (800-222-9932). These liquid combination homeopathic remedies work quickly, particularly on acute irritations that cause animals to be very uncomfortable and irritable.

- Rhus tox, a homeopathic remedy, for extremely irritated, red, and itchy skin.

- Kai Yeung, a Chinese herb, for clearing up chronic dermatitis marked by continuous irritation and either dry, flaking skin or skin clogged with a greasy material (seborrhea). The herb is available through Asia Herbs (415-989-9268).

- For general health and to give the skin extra nourishment, I suggest the regular use of a good multiple vitamin, mineral, and fatty acid supplement. My own formula, Daily Health Nuggets, is available through Earth Animal (800-711-2292).

DOSAGE

- **Vitamin B$_6$:** 25 milligrams twice daily with food. Give for seven to ten days, and then reduce dosage or eliminate as condition improves.

- **Skin and Seborrhea or Scratch Free:** Give 7 drops three times daily for three to four days. When incessant scratching has subsided and animal is calmer, give same number of drops twice a day for seven to ten more days. Then discontinue. Follow this procedure for any future flare-ups.

- **Rhus tox 6X:** 1 pellet or a few drops twice daily or as often as every two to three hours until you see improved appearance and less itching, usually by the end of the first day. Continue for one week.

- **Kai Yeung:** 1 caplet once a day, or twice if scratching is severe, for three to four weeks or until symptoms abate. Reduce dosage by half for the following month. Then discontinue.

- **Daily Health Nuggets:** Follow label instructions.

Herbs, Essences, Plus Supplement—Shannon Hines, DVM

For animals with dry, scaly, and itchy skin and poor hair coat, I recommend two helpful products. They can be used by themselves or, as I prefer, combined. One is Skin & Hair for Dogs, a liquid blend of herbs and flower essences made by Tasha's Herbs (800-315-0142). This formula helps to remove toxins and stimulate a healthy exterior. It contains burdock root, red clover, nettles, yellow dock, and red raspberry leaf and is laced with cold liver oil, vitamin E, and lecithin for palatability and extra nutrition.

The other product is Missing Link, made by Designing Health (800-774-7387), a whole-food nutritional supplement supplying important nutrients and enzymes for better skin and digestion.

DOSAGE
- Follow label instructions.

Make Your Own Healing Shampoo—Roger DeHaan, DVM

For a great antiseptic shampoo—that both kills fleas and soothes irritated skin—try this simple approach:

Add 10 drops of tea tree oil and a tablespoon of aloe vera into an 8 ounce bottle of your regular pet shampoo. Then, separately, add 1 tablespoon of apple cider vinegar to a pint of water.

Shampoo the animal as normal and let the shampoo stand for six to ten minutes. Rinse off well.

Then rinse again with the apple cider–spiked water. The purpose of this is to restore the natural pH of the skin. Dogs and cats have a slightly acidic skin. Most shampoos are somewhat alkaline. This difference many times leaves animals with irritated and itchy skin after shampooing. Rinsing with an apple cider vinegar solution after a shampoo often eliminates the problem.

⚜ Stress ⚜

See also Behavioral Problems

It may not be apparent to you, but stress could be causing your cat's health problem.

"Stress is too often the unrecognized problem behind the problem," says Toronto veterinarian Paul McCutcheon, DVM. "It can play a tremendous role in nearly every condition that a veterinarian treats."

Stress is a nonspecific reaction of the body to demands put on it. Reactions to demands are widely varied, from emotional disturbances to wear and tear of the system that contributes to illness. For us humans, stress could come in the form of not having enough money to pay the mortgage, difficulties on the job, or marital discord.

For an animal, stress can be brought on by boredom; an owner who doesn't provide enough attention, variety, or exercise; interpersonal relationships with members of the family or other animals in the household; and unpleasant environmental conditions. All of these factors start to add up and can undermine the immune system. As the burden of stress grows, the immune system becomes overworked, and the potential for problems increase. Chronic stress also impacts the adrenal glands, the body's stress organs. In time the adrenals may become exhausted, which lessens the animal's ability to deal with any new or continuing stress. Weakened adrenals also erode immune function.

Anything from skin problems to behavioral disorders can result from this simplified scenario. Unless you act to lessen the stress in the cat's life, a sick animal may not respond well to treatment, says McCutcheon.

Donna Starita Mehan, DVM, suggests evaluating the level of stress in your animal in the same manner that you would for people. She offers the following points:

- Is your animal relaxed or tense in its environment?
- Is your animal content or happy or constantly concerned or fearful that something is going to happen? Defensive, angry, or jealous?
- Is your animal suspicious of other animals and people or interacting with others well?
- Does your animal smile? Animals do smile.

"These are important considerations in assessing your animal's level of contentment—or lack of it," she says. "Remember that your level of physical health is dictated by your level of stress. If you have an animal who is easygoing, well balanced, interactive, and playful, that animal is going to be less prone to chronic illness. The mind/body connection applies to animals just as it applies to us."

McCutcheon, who routinely educates his clients about stress, tells pet owners to put themselves in their animal's place and consider possible sources of stress.

"Examine the animal's lifestyle and relationship with you, other people, or other animals in the household," he says. "Is there discord in your house? Stress in the household may very well be transmitted to the animals who live there. Is there a new addition or major change in the household that is affecting the pet? Are you spending more time away from home? If you take the time to look beneath the surface of symptoms, you will often find the real reason for the animal's stress. Then you can try to modify the situation in some way."

COMMON SIGNS OF STRESSED CATS

- Behavioral spraying, particularly the male.
- Reclusiveness or aggressiveness, depending on the individual.
- Chronic skin problems, itchiness around the face.
- Pica—eating of nonfood objects.
- Obesity and anorexia, which may be caused in part by stress.
- Urinary tract blockages. The major overlooked cause is stress. Stress affects the adrenal glands, which in turn affect the body's mineral balance, which in turn creates the conditions for the buildup of crystals and stones in the urinary tract.

What to Do About Stressed Pets—Paul McCutcheon, DVM

Here are some practical considerations for lowering the stress level in your animal's life:

- Feed a good diet, with as high-quality ingredients and as few chemical additives as possible. Poor-quality food can stress an animal's body.

- Consider the physical environment that you offer a pet. Is it reasonable for the animal? If you are about to choose an animal, try to match the surroundings to the animal.

- Cats need an outlet for their energy. They need to be stimulated with toys and activity.

- Avoid unnecessary medication. Drugs cover up symptoms and do not address root problems.

- In my practice I use homeopathic or Bach flower remedies to help stressed or anxious animals. The appropriate remedy depends on each individual situation. Many combination homeopathic and flower essence remedies are available in the marketplace, and you can try them on your own first. If they do not work, see an animal behaviorist or holistic veterinarian. And remember this important point: You may be able to calm down a stressed animal with a natural remedy, but you really want to locate and correct, if possible, the source of stress.

- When considering any healing program for your animal, do not overlook the possibility that stress may be contributing to the condition and that you may therefore need to deal with the stress to have a successful outcome.

St. John's Wort and Other Aids—Donna Starita Mehan, DVM

In severely stressed animals I have excellent results with St. John's Wort, the same herbal that has become very popular for people as a natural treatment for depression. For me it is the number one antianxiety, adrenal-supportive remedy. We see changes in a couple of days. It can be a lifesaver for animals by naturally reducing anxiety without causing drowsiness or suppression of mental activity. Persistent anxiety can lead to depression through adrenal and physical burnout.

The adrenal glands are intimately related to the nervous system. They are packed with nerve endings. If the adrenals become exhausted, the central nervous system will suffer. To protect the nervous system, I frequently use phenylalanine, an amino acid with a calming effect. This substance is regarded as a natural antidepressant and mood elevator. Phenylalanine contributes to a series of biochemical transformations that exert a strong and positive effect on mood and behavior, favoring a state of relaxation and increased mental activity.

Vitamins B_{12} and folic acid, two members of the B-complex vitamin family, are important nutrients for the normal functioning of the nervous system. I recommend these vitamins as well to help stressed animals.

St. John's Wort and phenylalanine can be purchased at the health food store. For B_{12} and folic acid, I use a combination called B_{12} Folic, made by Pure Encapsulations (800-753-CAPS; sold through health professionals). If you are not able to obtain this particular formula, pick up B_{12} and folic acid supplements at a health food store and follow the dosage suggestion below.

DOSAGE

- **St. John's wort:** 100 milligrams twice a day.

- **Phenylalanine:** 100 milligrams twice a day.

- **B$_{12}$ Folic:** Each capsule contains 800 micrograms of both nutrients. Give the equivalent of about 200 micrograms of each nutrient—1/4 capsule.

⋙ Surgery ⋘

Many holistic veterinarians recommend Arnica, a popular homeopathic remedy well-known for its ability to speed recovery from trauma, bruising, and surgery. Refer to chapter 9 on general guidelines for administering homeopathic medicines.

"There is much less scarring, stiffness, and soreness with Arnica," says Thomas Van Cise, DVM. "Many pet owners say their animals are back acting normally very soon. Even for serious surgery, Arnica speeds healing and helps animals rapidly get back up to full steam."

It is not necessary to give Arnica before surgery. Giving it before, as some people do, may create a need for somewhat more anesthesia.

"Give Arnica as soon as possible after surgery," says Van Cise. "I always stick a couple of Arnica 30C pellets right under the tongue of the anesthetized animal when surgery is completed."

Holistic veterinarians also frequently recommend variations of vitamins C and E and other nutrients to promote healing nutritionally.

BEFORE SURGERY

Milk Thistle for the Liver—Pamela Wood-Krzeminski, DVM

I routinely do a presurgical blood screening. If there is a mild elevation of liver enzymes, I recommend milk thistle on a daily basis for three or four weeks. Milk thistle is a magnificent herb for protecting and purifying the liver. A mild elevation of enzymes indicates some irritation or sluggishness in the liver. I prefer to have the liver operating maximally before it has to deal with the chemical onslaught of an anesthetic drug. I find that this short course of milk thistle noticeably improves the enzyme levels in more than half the cases. I use a milk thistle extract made by Twin Labs, available in health food stores.

DOSAGE
- 1 capsule daily. Empty the contents of the capsule in the animal's food.

Multivitamins—Wendell Belfield, DVM

Animals should be routinely maintained on a good multi-vitamin mineral supplement. If your animal is facing surgery in the immediate future and is not receiving a daily supplement, start supplementing well in advance of the procedure. This type of nutritional fortification enhances recovery and healing.

Rescue Remedy for Anxiety—Paul McCutcheon, DVM

To help relieve an animal's anxieties and fears, use the popular flower essence Rescue Remedy before surgery. It can be given several times during the day of the anticipated surgery. The animal will appear calmer and less anxious as an effect of the remedy.

Flower Remedy Combination—Jean Hofve, DVM

For the cat (or dog) facing major surgery or who has been diagnosed with a serious, long-term condition, I have had excellent results with Recuperation, a liquid flower remedy combination. The formula gives hope to the animal, marshals energy, and allows the animal to draw upon its own inner resources. It also works well for recovery from illness, injury, or surgery. The remedy can be purchased through the Internet from Flower Essence Therapy for Animals (http://home.earthlink.net/~jhofve).

The combination features Honeysuckle, for restoring depleted energy; Gentian for giving hope; and Sweet Chestnut for animals in despair. Flower remedies do not interfere with any medication. (For more information on flower remedies, and how to use them, see chapter 10.)

For surgical situations, start the remedy several days before the operation and then resume again as soon as you have the animal back home or as soon as your veterinarian will permit.

Recuperation is totally harmless. Many vets will "humor" an owner and allow the remedy to be given while the animal is in the hospital. It's worth making the request.

AFTER SURGERY

B Complex Plus Vitamin C Plus Amino Acids—Nino Aloro, DVM

A simple supplement program of B-complex vitamins, vitamin C, and amino acids helps speed healing and recovery. The B-complex product I use is Lipocaps, made by Vetus Animal Health and distributed by Burns Veterinary Supply (800-922-8767). Use any vitamin C product. The amino multi I recommend is Pure Form Amino Acids, from Jo-Mar Labs (800-538-4545).

If your animal isn't taking supplements regularly, start this program a week or at least several days before surgery and maintain it for a month afterward. Inform your veterinarian. These supplements do not interfere with the medical procedure or any medication.

DOSAGE
- **Lipocaps:** 1 capsule.

- **Vitamin C:** 250 milligrams daily; twice a day for larger cats.

- **Pure Form Amino Acids:** 2 capsules daily.

Speed Healing with Vitamins C and E—Nancy Scanlan, DVM

The simple addition of vitamins C and E to a cat's food after surgery is always helpful.

DOSAGE
- **Vitamin C:** 125 milligrams twice daily.

- **Vitamin E:** 50 IU once daily.

Arnica—Michele Yasson, DVM

I have seen some remarkable recoveries from surgery simply by using this great homeopathic remedy. Sutures sometimes can come out in half the normal time.

DOSAGE

- **Arnica 30C:** For minor procedures, such as dental treatment with one extraction, give twice a day following surgery for two days. After major surgeries give three times daily for four days, or longer if needed.

Make Your Own Arnica Formula—Paul McCutcheon, DVM

To encourage healing and relief from pain, try this homeopathic combination:

Drop 10 pellets each of Arnica 6X, Hypericum 6X, and Staphysagria 6X in 1 ounce of spring or filtered water. Give a half dropperful several times a day for several days, starting right after surgery.

Arnica is a well-known homeopathic remedy for bruising. Hypericum is beneficial for nerves, incisions, and pain. Staphysagria works on the level of deeper pain.

Arnica Plus Hypericum Plus Vitamin C—Charles Loops, DVM

The combination of the homeopathic remedies Arnica and Hypericum, along with vitamin C, has worked well to speed recovery of my patients. Hypericum is effective against pain.

DOSAGE

- **Arnica 30C and Hypericum 30C:** Alternate remedies hourly or every two hours the day after surgery. Decrease dosage over next several days.

- **Vitamin C:** 500 milligrams twice daily.

Phosphoricum to Curb Bleeding—Thomas Van Cise, DVM

The homeopathic remedy Phosphoricum acidum is an excellent aid against internal bleeding that may follow abdominal surgery or occur as a result of a traumatic event.

DOSAGE
• **Phosphoricum 12C:** Twice daily for two days.

Phosphorus for Postsurgical Vomiting—Jean Hofve, DVM

If you have an animal that is vomiting after surgery and can't keep food down, the homeopathic remedy Phosphorus works very well. Animals will sometimes be nauseated and vomit postoperatively as a reaction to the anesthesia. If the vomiting persists, contact your veterinarian.

DOSAGE
• **Phosphorus 30C:** 1 dose.

Topical Relief: Vitamin E and Magnets—Roger DeHaan, DVM

Prick a vitamin E capsule and apply the oil to the site of an incision. It will help speed the healing process at the site. If the animal licks the vitamin, no problem.

Magnets can accelerate healing. Use "flexi-pad," North Pole negative polarity or circular north-south magnets, but never a straight South Pole magnet. Apply the magnet to the surgery point for a minimum of twenty minutes at a time twice a day. If the animal is bandaged, you can slip it under the bandage. This will help against pain and inflammation and dramatically cut healing time, often in half. I obtain my magnets from Mid-America Marketing in Eaton, Ohio (800-922-1744).

⅏ Tooth Cavities ⅏

See Dental Health

Upper-Respiratory Infections

See Infectious Illnesses

Urinary Tract Problems

It used to be called feline urinary syndrome (FUS), and now the popular term is feline lower-urinary tract disease (FLUTD). Whatever you call it, urinary tract ailments affect a lot of cats, as many as 10 percent or more, according to veterinary studies.

Trouble develops in the bladder and/or the urethra, the narrow tube that carries urine out of the body, and basically appears in two forms:

1. Infections, generally caused by bacterial, fungal, or parasitic agents.
2. "Stones," comprising minerals, mucus, cellular debris, and other material, in the bladder or urethra. This problem is more dangerous for male cats because the sandy particles can partially or wholly plug up their urethras, which are narrower and longer than in females. An obstruction causes urine to back up into the body. Any blockage going on for more than five or six hours can be an emergency situation. A bladder can rupture, or a cat can become poisoned and die within twenty-four hours.

Although the causes of disease are varied, the signs are usually similar and dramatic—a cat straining and making repeated, prolonged attempts to pass urine. Sometimes only a few drops will spill. An affected cat is usually very uncomfortable and may be in a great deal of pain. See a veterinarian at once if this occurs. Conventional treatment can be very effective in a crisis and is necessary if a urinary obstruction is present.

Other signs may include the following:

- Licking the genital area excessively.
- Urinating outside the litter box.
- A cat spending a lot of time in the litter box.
- Blood in the urine.
- Lethargy.
- Hardly eating.
- Hunched for hours.
- Breath smelling of urine.

Years ago veterinary researchers believed they had found the answer to the problem of crystal formation by reducing the quantity of dietary minerals (the ash content), particularly magnesium. This finding set off a trend of low-ash diets among pet food manufacturers. In the mid-1980s research at the University of California at Davis overturned the ash theory. Investigators found that magnesium oxide, an alkaline compound, contributed to crystals when added to the diet, but when they switched to magnesium chloride, an acidic compound, crystals actually dissolved. It then became apparent that the presence of magnesium was not the cause of the crystal formation in the urine, but the pH of the urine was a factor. Under acidic conditions, the crystals dissolved. This finding in turn triggered another response from the manufacturers—acid-producing foods.

The results were good—and bad. Most of the typical urinary tract stones are made up of either magnesium ammonium phosphate (also known as struvite) or calcium oxalate. As a result of feeding the higher-acidic diets, the incidence of the alkaline struvite stones has indeed decreased, but there has been a disturbing increase in the incidence of calcium oxalate stones, which develop in a strongly acidic urine.

The solution to this dilemma, holistic veterinarians consistently point out, is to feed a cat the natural food it evolved on: raw meat. Cats in the wild don't develop this problem. They eat raw meat, which creates a naturally healthy level of acidic urine.

Holistic veterinarians often recommend acupuncture for chronic urinary tract infections. "Results are excellent," says Joseph Demers, DVM. "It is a very effective option for animals who have been on long-term antibiotics. With a few treatments, along with a good diet, we can achieve total remission in many cases or a significant reduction in the frequency of infections. When infections recur, a single acupuncture treatment generally resolves the problem. It works well also for nonbacterial infections."

Veterinarians find that stress can promote episodes of urinary tract disorders. You may not be aware of it, but stress can aggravate an existing condition and trigger a crisis. In one study, a change in weather and a move to a new environment were linked to the onset of urinary tract distress. A cat can be upset by its owner going on vacation, working longer hours for some period and not seeing an animal as much as usual, or by a big party in the house. If you suspect there may be a stress connection, see a veterinarian familiar with flower essences or homeopathy who can recommend the proper remedies for your individual animal.

"It is only slowly being recognized that the urinary system is highly susceptible to stress," says Roger DeHaan, DVM. "Cats bond strongly. Even aloof or independent cats, given a new owner, a new food, a new stress—may suddenly manifest blood in the urine. They miss us, the routine, the home, our voice. They may pretend they don't need us, then get sick when we leave them or send them off. They feel fearful and rejected and alone. Often in ways we do not readily understand, the human/cat bond can be incredibly strong."

THE WATER CONNECTION

It is critical for male cats with chronic urinary tract problems to drink enough water to keep them flushed out. The problem is how to encourage a cat to drink water. Nan Baumgartner, at the Village Veterinary Clinic in Oldenburg, Indiana, has found a technique that often works. "Crumble up fresh catnip in the cat's drinking water," she says. "The animal will often go wild for the taste and drink up quantities. Just a leaf or two is all that it takes. But it must be fresh. And you must crumble the leaves under the water and not just sprinkle the pieces on top. It doesn't work all the time, but when it does it can be a lifesaver."

Another water issue of potential importance to these cases relates to the alkalinity of your drinking water. In Lexington, Michigan, Lynne Friday, DVM, sees many cases of bladder stones and "gravel" in the urine, which she thinks has a good deal to do with the hard water in her local area. It has a high calcium carbonate content. "If you have a similar drinking water situation, you may want to put some apple cider vinegar in the water or food, or supplement the diet with vitamin C, which has a good preventive effect," she says.

HERBS

Ashwaganda for Stressed Cats—Tejinder Sodhi, DVM

A few years ago I was presented with a cat who suffered from recurrent bladder problems, specifically episodes of straining and passing blood in the urine. The cat had been on homeopathy, vitamin C, cranberry juice, and antibiotics, but nothing was working. After questioning the cat's owner, I realized that the problem was stress related. Friction within the household was causing the episodes of inflammatory bladder symptoms. I wanted a remedy that would have a calming as well as an anti-inflammatory effect. The answer was ashwaganda, a classic Indian herb with both these properties. The herb was right on target. The cat experienced no more recurrences. Subsequently I have used ashwaganda on nearly fifty similar cases with equally good results. The product I use is a liquid ashwaganda from Ayush Herbs (800-925-1371).

DOSAGE
- 10 drops per ten pounds of body weight twice daily. Use for up to two months to eliminate the inflammation, and then as needed.

HOMEOPATHIC REMEDIES

Remedies for Acute Episodes—Charles Loops, DVM

Homeopathic remedies work very well during the early stages of this condition before serious symptoms develop. You may even be able to avoid complete obstruction, and resolve the problem, with the appropriate acute remedy. The following remedies (in bold) and signs can help guide you to the right remedy to help avoid a severe episode:

- **Thlaspi bursa**—when there is blood and copious amounts of "sand" in the urine, burning urination, strong odor to urine, dribbling, straining.

- **Urtica urens**—blood in the urine, straining without urination, dribbling, retention of urine for long periods.
- **Coccus cacti**—swelling of penis, burning, itching, violent pain when urinating.
- **Cantharis**—retention of urine, cramping from bladder and with attempts at urination, frequent straining with dribbling, pus in the urine, burning pain with urination.
- **Colocynthus**—tense, very painful bladder, thick and gelatinous urine, fetid odor of urine, arched back with straining to urinate, burning after urination.
- **Apis mellifica**—burning pains, lack of thirst, swelling of urethra, frequent urging with only a few drops, and irritability.

In my practice I have been most successful with Urtica urens, Thlaspi bursa, Cantharis, and Apis mellifica. Keep a supply of remedies or a remedy kit at home for this condition. If symptoms arise, you need to administer the most appropriate remedy as soon as possible.

If, after trying remedies on your own, your cat continues to experience renewed episodes, I highly recommend that you consult a homeopathic veterinarian for constitutional treatment. This condition can become chronic and more difficult to cure, especially if repeated episodes are suppressed with allopathic drugs. Repeated treatment with the acute remedies recommended here may possibly lead to suppression as well because the cat requires a chronic, constitutional remedy.

To help with the healing process, I recommend vitamin C plus parsley water as a diuretic once the cat is urinating normally.

Dosage
- Use a remedy with potencies below 30C—that is, 6X or C, 12X or C, or 30X. If symptoms are severe, such as repeated straining or pain, give a dose of the selected remedy every fifteen minutes. If you do not see an improvement after several doses, try the next most indicated remedy and use it the same way. If the situation continues or worsens, see a veterinarian immediately. If improvement occurs after a few doses, continue administering the remedy for several more doses. Then wait a few hours between doses, unless the symptoms recur

sooner. If you are in doubt, contact a homeopathic veterinarian or take your cat to be examined. If you are going to be giving several doses of a particular remedy over a short period of time, place a pellet or two in 1/2 ounce of distilled water, let them dissolve, and use a few drops of this liquid for each dose.

- **Vitamin C:** 500 milligrams twice daily.

NUTRITIONAL SUPPLEMENTS

Methionine to Acidify Urine—Nancy Scanlan, DVM

Many cats with urinary tract problems have alkaline urine. Simply by acidifying the urine *slightly*, you may be able to improve and sometimes eliminate the problem. One easy way to do this is to add methionine, an amino acid, right into the food.

First check the urine. Your veterinarian can do it for you or you can check it yourself using a simple litmus paper test. You probably remember using litmus paper in high school chemistry. You can purchase litmus strips through science, laboratory, or chemical supply stores, or ask your local pharmacist. The small strips determine the acidity or alkalinity of a substance. Pink is acid. Blue is alkaline. Lavender is in between. You want to make the urine *slightly* on the acidic side, so lavender to pink is the desired color. Simply place a strip in the litter box sand where the cat has just urinated. If the strip indicates the urine is neutral or alkaline, than start the methionine. You want to make the urine *slightly* on the acidic side.

Always be sure to check the urine first before doing this. If your animal is already on a special acidifying diet, the urine may be acidic enough and you don't want to increase the acidity. However, some diets that claim to acidify the urine don't work.

If you see an animal straining for several days and only a few drops come out each time, you can wait a couple of days after starting the methionine supplement to see if it works. If you have any doubts, see your veterinarian right away. Do not use this procedure if your cat already has oxalate stones, which occur in acidic urine.

DOSAGE

- 100 milligrams twice daily, or three times if necessary. Check the urine level again in a few days. If the level is not yet slightly acidic, go to the third dose. If you give too much methionine, an animal will throw up, but for most cases this is a very safe range.

Vitamin C for Relief—Mark Haverkos, DVM

If you put cats on vitamin C at the early stages of this, and keep them on it, you can often avoid future problems and medical bills. Frequency of urination and straining are signs to bring on vitamin C if you haven't already done so. I recommend Ester C or sodium ascorbate (nonacidic vitamin C).

DOSAGE
- Small and medium-size cats, 250 milligrams two times a day; large cats, 500 milligrams two times a day. Crunch up a tablet or mix powder right into the food.

FOOD AND SPECIAL DIETS

Stop the Dry Food and Nibbling—Michele Yasson, DVM

Stop the dry food. It's a must! Dry food is an absolute obstacle to cure. I am able to resolve about half of my cases just by having the owner switch to a canned food or a wetter food.

Feed once or twice a day. Don't allow cats to nibble. After meals there is an alkaline tide that occurs in the body. In the bladder, alkaline urine tends to create crystals from the dissolved minerals. Dry food means a greater concentration of minerals. Allowing animals to nibble throughout the day means a prolongation of the alkaline tide.

Among the cats who have responded to the diet change alone were animals who had several previous episodes and had been catheterized by other veterinarians. They included male cats facing possible surgical removal of the penis in order to prevent future plugging of the narrow urethra. Often a male cat with this condition will plug up at the tip of the urethra. Even though a drastic step, surgery is sometimes recommended because a blocked urethra is a life-threatening situation. Female cats have a wider urethra and are able to pass crystals out more easily.

Another important step you can take is to institute a twenty-four-hour fast once a week whenever you see your cat straining or visiting the litter box often. The fast will reduce the influx of minerals in the body and also put the body in a healing mode. Instead of expending energy on digesting food, the body thus diverts attention to restoring balance throughout the system, including the urinary tract. Be sure the cat has access to plenty of water.

Real Meat Plus Supplements—Jean Hofve, DVM

Animals eating natural food diets, and more wet food, are less likely to develop this condition. Most commercial cat foods contain chemical acidifiers as a preventive. Some prescription diets recommended for cats with a history of FUS are so acidic that if an animal eats these types of foods long enough, they run the risk of developing calcium oxalate crystals that have to be removed surgically. I recently operated on a cat that had been on c/d prescription diet for eight years. The cat never had a problem to begin with, but years before, the cat's brother had had an FUS condition and the veterinarian had prescribed the special diet. The owner figured it was easier to feed both cats the same food and did so for years. The cat I was now asked to treat was plugged. I removed forty tiny stones from that cat! This is a whole new problem that has never before been seen in cats. Diets like c/d shouldn't be fed long-term. They are good in a crisis, but don't use them longer than a couple of months.

The best thing to do is feed the cats meat. That accomplishes the same thing—lowering the urine pH—in a natural way. Leaving food out all day may also contribute to FUS. Each time an animal nibbles, the pancreas excretes bicarbonate into the system, and this may elevate the alkaline level.

Cats need real meat, not ersatz by-products. Meat naturally acidifies the urine and prevents the buildup of alkalinity and the potential for problems in the bladder.

I have tried many different supplements and remedies for this condition depending on the individual situation. The ones I like the best are these:

- CoenzymeQ$_{10}$ (CoQ$_{10}$, for short), a popular and effective antioxidant and energizer. CoQ$_{10}$ is actually a fat-soluble vitamin that is better absorbed when taken with fat.

- Cranberry is a traditional natural remedy. We don't know exactly how it works, but it indeed helps. It probably acidifies the urine to counteract the alkaline buildup. I use a supplement called Cranacton, a product sold at health food stores.

DOSAGE
- **CoQ$_{10}$:** 10 milligrams daily for a week to ten days after a crisis. Thereafter for maintenance, 5 milligrams a day per each ten pounds of body weight. Mix into food, or give it with some kind of fatty food that the cat will like.
- **Cranacton:** 1 capsule a day, half in the morning and half at night, during an acute flare-up. Mix it in with smelly food because cats usually don't like the taste.

Wet Food Plus Chinese Herbs—Joseph Demers, DVM

In Chinese medicine, urinary tract infections are called "damp heat" conditions. If you feed dry food to an animal with this condition, you are creating more heat in the body. If there is already a weakness in the bladder, guess where the buildup of additional heat occurs? In a matter of months there is another urinary tract infection.

The number one preventive action you can take is getting off dry food. Give the urinary tract more moisture. Cats don't drink much water, so the way to get more moisture into their bodies is to feed them raw meat or canned food or add broth to their dry food.

I use an excellent Chinese herbal formula known as Te Xiao Pai Shi Wan, or, in English, Specific Drug Passwan. The product is available in Chinese pharmacies or groceries. If you have difficulty locating it, contact a veterinary acupuncturist who uses Chinese herbal medicine.

This natural medicine is designed to eliminate the "damp heat" and counteract crystallization, where stones or "gravel" are present in the kidneys, bladder, or urethras. Typical of many Chinese herbals, this remedy comes in the form of tiny black pills. The major ingredients are lysimachia leaf, lygopodium fungus, and angelica root.

The formula is very helpful for situations where your cat is straining to urinate and every few minutes returns to the litter box and manages only a few drops, or where you see signs of sandy, gravel-like material in the urine. Within a day or two of starting the remedy, you are likely to notice more comfortable urination as the formula goes to work in the body. This is a product that has a tonifying effect on the urinary tract and can be used long-term in case an animal is prone to recurrent problems.

DOSAGE
- 2 or 3 pills twice a day, generally for ten days. If the cat has a history of recurrences, give the formula for a month and then for ten days every two or three months. Smear the tiny pills with butter to give them a palatable taste and help slide them down the throat.

Cranberry Formula #1—Wendell Belfield, DVM

I have found a simple solution to acidify the urine and dissolve crystals in cats with recurrent obstruction problems. These are animals who have lost the ability to maintain the acidic level necessary to keep the crystals in solution. My remedy is Carpon, an extract of cranberry in tablet form (available through Orthomolecular Specialties at 408-227-9334). A high-level, good-quality protein diet in combination with the extract works excellently. Dissolution of crystals can be expected within twenty-four hours. Cats may remain on this program indefinitely with no adverse effects.

DOSAGE
- For an average-size cat, use one 250-milligram tablet twice daily for five days. Afterward the cat can be maintained on a single tablet daily. For larger cats, use 2 tablets twice daily in the beginning and then reduce the dosage to 2 once a day. Either put the tablet down the cat's throat or mix it into wet food.

Cranberry Formula #2—Pedro Luis Rivera, DVM

Cranberry Comfort, a product containing cranberry along with other natural ingredients, has given me great results with chronic urinary tract infections that are unresponsive to conventional treatment with antibiotics. The product is available through NaturVet at 888-628-8793. The cranberry helps to minimize bacterial colonization of the bladder mucosa. The formula also contains marshmallow root, Oregon grapeseed, and vitamin C to help control inflammation. Echinacea is added to help boost the immune system.

DOSAGE
• Follow label instructions.

⚕ Vomiting ⚕

See Digestive Disorders

⚕ Yeast Infections ⚕

See also Digestive Disorders, Ear Problems, and Skin Disorders and Allergies

Yeast infections are rampant conditions that stem from an imbalance of the bacteria population of the intestines. They often manifest in these ways:

• Itchy skin.
• Itchy toes and a reddish black discoloration between the toes that has an odor like smelly gym socks.
• Digestive disorders.
• Chronic itchy ears, particularly if there is a reddish black discharge.

"Be careful with the ears," cautions Donna Starita Mehan, DVM. "Some cases may involve ear mites. Ear mites show up as a clumpy, grayish black granular discharge. Sometimes you can see the tiny white mites crawling around in this debris. By comparison, a yeast infection will smell yeasty and have a greasy, reddish black color to it."

Adds Karen Bentley, DVM: "Many ear problems are yeast based.

If there is a chronic combination of ear and skin problems, suspect a yeast infection. Most of the time, the animal has had a history of antibiotics."

Holistic veterinarians frequently treat yeast infections that have developed after antibiotics or vaccinations and a resultant depression of the immune system.

"Conventional veterinary treatments can often be a cause of yeast infections," Mehan points out. "If you bring in an animal for treatment with itchy skin or a bowel upset, a veterinarian will often prescribe an antibiotic. This will further upset the digestive tract, and then you have new problems—a 'double whammy.' In my practice, yeast infections are more often involved in digestive disorders than any other cause, including parasites."

Probiotics and Vinegar Vs. Yeast—Donna Starita Mehan, DVM

A major weapon against yeast infections is a probiotic supplement containing billions of beneficial bacteria, such as acidophilus, that can restore proper bacterial balance in the intestines. I also suggest adding and mixing in a small amount of nonpasteurized apple cider vinegar to the animal's food or water. Yeast do not grow well in an acid environment.

A large number of other products are designed to help balance the bowels in a healthy manner. See your holistic veterinarian for guidance, as you need to match the products to the specific requirements of the patient. It's also important to eliminate foods, such as wheat, sugar, and yeast, which tend to encourage the growth of yeast in the body.

DOSAGE
- **Probiotic:** If you use a human product, calculate the dose according to the animal's size.

- **Apple cider vinegar:** 1/8 teaspoon two times daily.

Grapefruit Seed Extract Plus Enzymes—Karen Bentley, DVM

I have had good results using a combination of grapefruit seed extract along with Feline Digestive Enzymes, from Dr. Goodpet (800-222-9932). Improvements are usually seen within two to three months. Both supplements should be taken long-term, for at least six months to a year, if the problem is long-standing. Be sure the animal is eating a high-quality diet and taking a good multi-vitamin/mineral supplement.

DOSAGE

- **Grapefruit seed extract:** one 100-milligram capsule three times a day.

- **Feline Digestive Enzymes:** Follow label instructions.

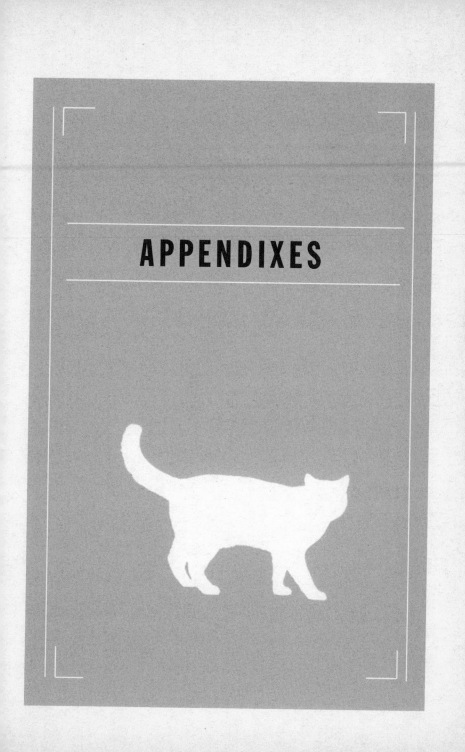

APPENDIXES

APPENDIX A

LIST OF CONTRIBUTING VETERINARIANS

The veterinarians whose names are listed in this section made this book possible by sharing their precious expertise with the author. Behind each name you will see the initials DVM or VMD, which are abbreviations meaning doctor of veterinary medicine.

Listed with each veterinarian are his or her special interests. Many of the veterinarians offer integrated medical services—that is, they perform surgery and prescribe medication in addition to their holistic specialties. Some also offer telephone consultation.

- Nino Aloro, DVM, Aloro Pet Clinic, 2212 Laskin Rd., Virginia Beach, VA 23454. Phone: 757-340-5040. Herbs and nutrition.

- Wendell O. Belfield, DVM, Bel-Mar Veterinary Hospital, 3091 Monterey Rd., San Jose, CA 95111. Phone: 408-227-9944. Ortho-molecular medicine, nutrition. Web site: www.belfield.com.

- Jan Bellows, DVM, All Pets Dental Clinic, 9111 Taft St., Pembroke Pines, FL 33024. Phone: 954-432-1111. Dental and general veterinary medicine. Web site: www.dentalvet.com.

- Karen Bentley, DVM, 1 Simcoe St., Guelph, Ontario, Canada N1E 3B7. Phone: 519-821-8859. Homeopathy, nutrition, herbal medicine, magnetic therapy.

- Carolyn S. Blakey, DVM, Westside Animal Clinic, 1831 West Main St., Richmond, IN 47374. Phone: 765-966-0015. Acupuncture, nutrition, homeopathy, herbs, flower remedies.

- Ron Carsten, DVM, Birch Tree Animal Hospital, 1602 Grand Ave., Glenwood Springs, CO 81601. Phone: 970-945-0125. Acupuncture, chiropractic, homeopathy, nutrition.

- Christina Chambreau, DVM, 908 Cold Bottom Rd., Sparks, MD 21152. Phone: 410-771-4968. Homeopathy.

- Roger DeHaan, DVM, 33667 Peace River Ranch Rd., Frazee, MN 56544-8818. Phone: 218-846-9112. Acupuncture, chiropractic, nutrition, homeopathy, herbs, magnetic therapy. Web site: www.aholisticvet.com.

- Joseph Demers, DVM, Holistic Animal Clinic, 496 North Harbor City Blvd., Melbourne, FL 32935. Phone: 407-752-0140. Acupuncture, homeopathy, herbs, Chinese medicine.

- Edmund R. Dorosz, DVM, P.O. Box 2094, Fort MacLeod, Alberta, Canada T0L 0Z0. Phone: 403-553-4140. Nutrition. Web site: www.ourpets.com.

- Lynne M. Friday, DVM, Lexington Veterinary Clinic, 5346 Main St., Lexington, MI 48450. Phone: 810-359-8828. Acupuncture, chiropractic, applied kinesiology, flower essences, homeopathy, herbs, nutrition.

- Maria Glinski, DVM, Silver Spring Animal Wellness Center, 1405 W. Silver Spring Dr., Glendale, WI 53209. Phone: 414-228-7655. Acupuncture, Chinese herbs, homeopathy, nutrition.

- Robert Goldstein, VMD, Northern Skies Veterinary Center, Westport, CT 06880. Phone: 203-222-0260. Nutrition.

- Stan Gorlitsky, DVM, Shem Creek Animal Hospital, 461 Coleman Blvd., Mt. Pleasant, SC 29464. Phone: 843-881-9915. Acupuncture, homeopathy, nutrition, herbs.

- Mark Haverkos, DVM, Village Veterinary Clinic, P.O. Box 119, 22163 Main St., Oldenburg, IN 47036. Phone: 812-934-2410. Acupuncture, chiropractic, nutrition, herbs, homeopathy.

- Shannon Hines, DVM, Orchard Animal Clinic, 3305 S. Orchard Dr., Bountiful, UT 84010. Phone: 801-296-1230. Nutrition, homeopathy, chiropractic.

- Jean Hofve, DVM, P.O. Box 22302, Sacramento, CA 95822. Currently involved in animal advocacy work. Not in active practice. Nutrition, flower remedies, homeopathy. Web site: www.spirit-essence.com.

- A. Greig Howie, DVM, Dover Animal Clinic, 1151 S. Governors Ave., Dover, DE 19901. Phone: 302-674-1515. Acupuncture, nutrition, Chinese herbs, homeopathy.

- Jody Kincaid, DVM, Anthony Animal Clinic, 901 E. Franklin, Anthony, TX 79821. Phone: 915-886-4558. Acupuncture, herbs, nutrition.

- Charles Loops, DVM, 38 Waddell Hollow Rd., Pittsboro, NC 27312. Phone: 919-542-0442. Homeopathy.

- Paul McCutcheon, DVM, East York Animal Clinic, 805 O'Connor Dr., Toronto, Ontario, Canada M4B 2S7. Phone: 416-757-3569. Bach flowers, nutrition, homeopathy.

- Donna Starita Mehan, DVM, A Country Way Veterinary Care, 27728 S.E. Haley Rd. Boring, OR 97009. Phone: 503-663-7277. Herbs, nutrition, chiropractic, electroacupuncture, homeopathy, magnetic therapy, flower essences.

- Alfred J. Plechner, DVM, California Animal Hospital, 1736 S. Sepulveda, Los Angeles, CA 90025. Phone: 310-473-0960. Nutrition, endocrine-immune dysfunction.

- William Pollak, DVM, Fairfield Animal Hospital, 1115 E. Madison Ave., Fairfield, IA 52556. Phone: 515-472-6983. Nutrition, herbs, homeopathy, Ayurveda. Web site: www.healthyvet.com.

- Nancy Scanlan, DVM, Sherman Oaks Veterinary Group, 13624 Moorpark St., Sherman Oaks, CA 91423. Phone: 818-784-9977. Acupuncture, flower essences, Chinese herbs, nutrition, homeopathy, chiropractic. Web site: hibridge.com.

- Allen Schoen, DVM, Veterinary Institute for Therapeutic Alternatives, 15 Sunset Terrace, Sherman, CT 06784. Phone: 203-354-2287. Acupuncture, chiropractic, herbs, Chinese medicine, nutrition.

- Tejinder Sodhi, DVM, Animal Wellness Center, 2115 112th N.E. #100, Bellevue, WA 98208; and 6501 196th St., Lynnwood, WA 98036. Phone: 425-455-8900. Ayurveda, homeopathy, nutrition.

- Carvel Tiekert, DVM, Animal Clinic of Harford County, 2214 Old Emmorton Rd., Bel Air, MD 21015. Phone: 410-569-7777. Acupuncture, chiropractic, nutrition, homeopathy, applied kinesiology.

- Thomas E. Van Cise, DVM, All Animals Exotic or Small Hospital, 1560 Hamner Ave., Norco, CA 91760. Phone: 909-737-1242. Acupuncture, chiropractic, homeopathy, herbs.

- Pamela Wood-Krzeminski, DVM, VCA Boca Del Mar Animal Hospital, 7076 Bera Casa Way, Boca Raton, FL 33433. Phone: 561-395-4668. Nutrition, acupuncture, herbs, flower essences.

- Susan G. Wynn, DVM, Greater Atlanta Veterinary Medical Group, 1080 North Cobb Pkwy., Marietta, GA 30062. Phone: 770-424-6303. Acupuncture, herbs, homeopathy, nutrition. Web site: www.altvetmed.com.

- Michele Yasson, DVM, Holistic Veterinary Services, 1101 Route 32, Rosendale, NY 12472. Phone: 914-658-3923. Homeopathy, acupuncture, herbs, nutrition.

APPENDIX B

RESOURCES

Veterinary Organizations

- American Holistic Veterinary Medical Association, 2214 Old Emmorton Rd., Bel Air, MD 21015. Phone: 410-569-0795. Fax: 410-569-2346. E-mail: AHVMA@compuserve.com.

  Contact the association for the name and number of holistic veterinarians in your area. This flagship organization publishes the *Quarterly Journal of the American Holistic Veterinary Medical Association* available for $65 per year.

- The Academy for Veterinary Homeopathy, 1283 Lincoln St., Eugene, OR 97401. Phone: 541-342-7665. The AVH provides training in classical homeopathy for veterinarians, leading to certification. For the names of veterinarians who practice homeopathy, refer to the Internet Web site http://www.acadvethom.org or call 305-652-1590. The list is maintained by Miami veterinarian Larry Bernstein, VMD.

- International Veterinary Acupuncture Society, P.O. Box 1478, Longmont, CO 80502. Phone: 303-449-7936.

- American Veterinary Chiropractic Association, 623 Main St., Hillsdale, IL 61257. Phone: 309-658-2920. Fax: 309-658-2622.

Internet Web Sites of Interest

- Alternative Veterinary Medicine on the Internet: www.altvetmed.com. This supreme Internet Web site is the labor of love of Jan Bergeron, DVM, and Susan Wynn, DVM. It features a state-by-state directory of holistic veterinarians that enables you to quickly look up the nearest practitioner near you. You will also find excellent articles here on important pet health issues and conditions written by Wynn. Other features: alternative medicine resources, books and book suppliers, periodicals, and a list of premium natural pet foods.

- Critter Chatter: www.nwga.com/members/crchat. This excellent Web site is a full plate of information on breeding, shelters, rescues, pet food, diseases, people's experiences with veterinary drugs, veterinary commentaries, and even a chat room for kids to talk about pets.

- The Dog and Cat Book Catalog: www.dogandcatbooks.com. This Web site is loaded with hundreds of book and video titles on training and behavior, breeds, natural health and healing, pet loss, traveling with pets, grooming, kennel and cattery management, and even pet-sitting. If you don't have access to the Internet, call 1-800-776-2665 for a catalog.

Newsletters

- Robert and Susan Goldstein's *Love of Animals*. This jam-packed monthly gem of information is written by a pioneer holistic veterinarian and his wife, an expert on animal nutrition and behavior. Contains reader-friendly commentary on latest developments in veterinary medicine, regular ratings, analyses and recommendations on food, creative recipes, and a cornucopia of nutritional and natural care product tips. Published by Earth Animal LLC, 372 Danbury Rd., P.O. Box 809, Wilton, CT 06897-0809. Phone: 800-211-6365. Subscriptions: $69 per year.

Special Services

- The endocrine-immune imbalance blood test. National Veterinary Diagnostic Services, 23361 El Toro Rd., Suite 218, Lake Forest, CA 92630-6929. Phone: 949-859-3648.

- Bio-Nutritional Analysis. Robert Goldstein, VMD, Bioanalytics, Inc., Westport, CT, 06880. Phone: 800-670-0830.

- Seminars on Holistic Health and Homeopathy for Animals, Christina Chambreau, DVM, 908 Cold Bottom Rd., Sparks, MD 21152. E-mail: cbctina@aol.com.

- Natural Breeders Association, Marina Zacharias, P.O. Box 1436, Jacksonville, OR 97530. Phone: 541-899-2080. This organization publishes newsletters and directories for breeders and animal aficionados "who care and pride themselves in the health of their animals...special people who have chosen to learn and incorporate natural health care methods for their animals."

Manufacturers, Distributors, and Stores

Some of the companies listed below sell products only through health professionals, in which case you will have to ask your veterinarian or a licensed practitioner to purchase product for you. Some manufacturers and distributors can help you locate individual stores in your area that carry the products you want.

Animal Nutrition, Inc. (Pat McKay)
Food, supplements, books
396 W. Washington Blvd.
Pasadena, CA 91103
626-296-1120
800-975-7555 (orders only)
Web site:
home1.gte.net/patmckay/
index.html

Animal's Apawthecary
Herbs
P.O. Box 212
Conner, MT 59827
406-821-4090

Ayush Herbs, Inc.
Ayurvedic herbals
2115 112th Ave. N.E.
Bellevue, WA 98004
800-925-1371

Azmira Holistic Animal Care
Nutritional supplements,
neutraceutical, pet food
2100 N. Wilmot Rd. #109
Tucson, AZ 85712
800-497-5665
Web site: www.azmira.com

BHI Homeopathics
11600 Cochiti S.E.
Albuquerque, NM 87123
800-621-7644

Bio Vet International
Dismutase
5152 Bolsa Ave. #101
Huntington Beach, CA 92649
800-788-1084

Celestial Pets
9875 Gloucester Dr.
Beverly Hills, CA 90210
1-888-CEL PETS

Coastside Bio Resources
Sea cucumber supplements
P.O. Box 151
Stonington, ME 04681
207-367-2297

Designing Health Inc.
Nutritional supplements
28310 Ave. Crocker Unit G
Valencia, CA 91355
800-774-7387

Dr. Doolittle
A Health Food Store for Pets
572 Dundas St.
London, Ontario, Canada N6B
1W8
519-642-1130
888-CHEESIE
Web site: www.drdoo.com

Dr. Goodpet
Homeopathic remedies for
animals, nutritional supplements,
digestive enzymes, shampoo, stain
control garments
P.O. Box 4547
Inglewood, CA 90309
800-222-9932
Web site: www.goodpet.com

Earth Animal
Retail store and distributor natural
pet health care products
606 Post Rd. East
Westport, CT 06880
203-222-7173
800-711-2292

Emerson Ecologics
Nutritional supplements
18 Lomar Park
Pepperell, MA 01463
800-654-4432

Flower Essence Society
Flower essences
P.O. Box 459
Nevada City, CA 95959
800-736-9222
Web site: www.flowersociety.org

Flower Essence Therapy for
Animals
Flower essences
P.O. Box 22302
Sacramento, CA 95822
Web site:
www.spiritessence.com

Gaia Herbs, Inc.
12 Lancaster Country Rd.
Harvard, MA 01451
800-831-7780

Good Communications, Inc.
Nutritional supplements
P.O. Box 10069
Austin, TX 78766
800-968-1738

Green Foods Corporation
Barley Dog and Barley Cat
320 N. Graves Ave.
Oxnard, CA 93030
800-222-3374

Green Hope Farms
Flower essences
P.O. Box 125
Meriden, NH 03770
603-469-3662

Halo, Purely For Pets
Nutritional supplements, herbal
dips, herbal eye wash
3438 East Lake Rd. #14
Palm Harbor, FL 34685
800-426-4256

Hanna Kroeger Herbs
Hanna's Herb Shop
5684 Valmont
Boulder, CO 80301
800-206-6722

Health Concerns
Chinese herbal formulas
8001 Capwell Dr.
Oakland, CA 94621
800-233-9355

Holistic Pet Center
A health food store for pets
15599 S.E. 82nd Dr.
Clackamas, OR 97015
800-788-PETS
Web site:
www.holisticpetcenter.com

HomeoPet
Homeopathic remedies for animals
P.O. Box 147
Westhampton Beach, NY 11978
800-434-0449

Jo-Mar Labs
Nutritional supplements
251 "B" E. Hacienda
Campbell, CA 95008
800-538-4545

Morrill's New Directions
Natural pet health care products
P.O. Box 30
Orient, ME 04471
800-368-5057
Web site: www.morrills.com

Mt. Capra Cheese
Capra Mineral Whey
279 S.W. 9th St.
Chehalis, WA 98532
800-574-1961

Natural Animal Nutrition (NAN)
Nutritional supplements,
shampoos, pet food
2109 "A" Columbia Park Dr.
Edgewood, MD 21040
800-548-2899

Natural Pet Care Company
Retail store, mail order: food,
supplements, and remedies
8050 Lake City Way
Seattle, WA 98115
800-962-8266

NaturVet
Nutritional/neutraceutical
supplements
27461-B Diaz Rd.
Temecula, CA 92590
888-628-8783

New Action Products
Nutritional supplements
145 Ontario St.
Buffalo, NY 14207
716-873-3738

Newton Labs
Homeopathic remedies
2360 Rockaway Ind. Blvd.
Conyers, GA 30012
800-448-7256

NF Formulas
Nutritional supplements
805 S.E. Sherman
Portland, OR 97214
800-547-4891

Noah's Ark
Nutritional supplements
6166 Taylor Rd. #105
Naples, FL 34109
800-926-5100

Nutramax Laboratories
Neutraceutical products
5024 Campbell Blvd.
Baltimore, MD 21230
800-925-5187
Web site: www.nutramaxlabs.com

Orthomolecular Specialties
Nutritional supplements
3091 Monterey Rd.
San Jose, CA 95111-3204
408-227-9334

Pacific BioLogic
Chinese herbal formulas
P.O. Box 520
Clayton, CA 94517
800-869-8783

Perfect Health Diet (PHD)
Pet food
65 Court St.
White Plains, NY 10602
800-PHD-1502

Pet's Friend
Nutritional supplements, digestive
enzymes
5871 N. University Dr., Suite 720
Tamarac, FL 33321
954-720-0794
800-868-1009 (orders only)

PetSage
Natural pet health care products
and books
4313 Wheeler Ave.
Alexandria, VA 22304
800-PET-HLTH
Web site: www.petsage.com

Pets, Naturally
Retail store for holistic pet
products
13459 Ventura Blvd.
Sherman Oaks, CA 91423
818-784-1233

Professional Health Products
Manufactures/distributes
homeopathics, herbals, glandulars,
and supplements through health
professionals
211 Overlook Dr.
Sewickley, PA 15143
800-929-4133

Progressive Laboratories
1701 W. Walnut Hills Ln.
Irving, TX 75038
800-527-9512

Prozyme Products, Ltd.
Digestive enzymes
6600 N. Lincoln Ave.
Lincolnwood, IL 60645
800-522-5537

Pure Encapsulations
Nutritional supplements
490 Boston Post Rd.
Sudbury, MA 01776
800-753-CAPS

Quantum Herbal Products
Flea and tick repellents
20 Dewitt Dr.
Saugerties, NY 12477
800-348-0398

Seroyal International Inc
Nutritional supplements
44 E. Beaver Creek Rd. #17
Richmond Hill, Ontario, Canada
L4B 1G8
800-263-5861

Seven Forests Chinese Herbs
Available through I.T.M.
2017 S.E. Hawthorne
Portland, OR 97214
800-544-7504

Sojourner Farms
Pet food and nutritional
supplements
11355 Excelsior Blvd.
Hopkins, MN 55343
800-TO-SOJOS
Web site: www.sojos.com

Solid Gold Health Products for
Pets
Pet food and nutritional
supplements
1483 N. Cuyamaca
El Cajon, CA 92020
800-364-4863
Web site: http://www.solid-gold-
inc.com

St. Jon's—VRX Pharmaceuticals
St. Jon's sold over-the-counter;
VRX through veterinarians
Dental chews, natural toothpastes,
dentifrices, toothbrushes
1656 W. 240th St.
Harbor City, CA 90710
310-326-2720

Standard Process
Nutritional supplements sold
through health professionals
1200 W. Royal Lee Dr.
Palmyra, WI 53156
800-848-5061

Tasha's Herbs
P.O. Box 9888
Jackson, WY 83002
800-315-0142

Terra Oceana
Nutritional supplements
1187 Coast Village Rd. #485
Santa Barbara, CA 93108
805-563-2634

Tyson Neutraceuticals
Amino acids and nutritional
formulations
12832 Chadron Ave.
Hawthorne, CA 90250
800-318-9766

VetriScience Labs
Nutritional supplements sold
through veterinarians
20 New England Dr.
Essex Junction, VT 05453
800-882-9993

Whiskers Holistic Pet Products
Retail store and distributor of food
and natural health care products
235 E. 9th St.
New York, NY 10003
212-979-2532
800-WHISKERS (orders only)
Web site: choicemall.com/whiskers

Winter Sun Trading Co.
Western wild-crafted and organic
herbs and herbal books
107 N. San Francisco St. Suite 1
Flagstaff, AZ 86001
520-774-2884
Web site: www.wintersun.com

Wow-Bow Distributors
Natural pet health care products
13B Lucon Dr.
Deer Park, NY 11729
800-326-0230

APPENDIX C

RECOMMENDED READING

- *Complementary and Alternative Veterinary Medicine: Principles and Practice*, edited by Allen M. Schoen, DVM, and Susan G. Wynn, DVM (Mosby, 1998). This 820-page whopper is the first real textbook to cover in depth a wide variety of holistic approaches in veterinary medicine. Chapters are written by veterinarians and other experts. You'll find detailed information on nutrition, supplements, Chinese medicine, acupuncture, chiropractic, massage therapy, bioenergetic medicine, magnetic therapy, botanical medicine including Chinese, Ayurvedic, and Western herbs, homeopathy, aromatherapy, and flower remedy therapy and str]ategies for integrating holistic methods into conventional practices. Although the book is intended more for professional consumption, the "serious" layperson will find it a treasure of information. One of many books available through the American Holistic Veterinary Medical Association (410-569-0795).

- *Dr. Pitcairn's Complete Guide to Natural Health for Dogs and Cats*, by Richard H. Pitcairn, DVM, Ph.D., and Susan Hubble Pitcairn (Rodale Press), available in many book and health food stores. This is the gold standard book that even many veterinarians use for reference.

- *Pet Allergies: Remedies for an Epidemic*, by Alfred Plechner, DVM, and Martin Zucker (Very Healthy Enterprises, Inglewood, CA), available at 800-222-9932. This eye-opening book explains why dogs and cats get sick and die before their time and why there is a massive incidence of allergies among pets. It offers important solutions, such as the use of diet, digestive enzymes, trace minerals, and blood tests to determine endocrine-immune imbalances. The book was written in 1986, and according to Plechner, the epidemic has grown worse. A critical book for understanding problems that are sickening and killing many purebred animals and, increasingly, affecting mixed breeds as well.

- *Food Pets Die For: Shocking Facts About Pet Food*, by Ann Martin (NewSage Press, P.O. Box 607, Troutdale, OR 97060; phone: 503-695-2211). The title says it all.

- *The Very Healthy Cat Book*, by Wendell O. Belfield, DVM, and Martin Zucker, available through Orthomolecular Specialties, P.O. Box

32232, San Jose, CA 95152, 408-227-9334. This reprint of the original McGraw-Hill nutritional classic showcases the many benefits of vitamin and mineral supplementation, and particular of vitamin C, for cats.

- *Love, Miracles and Animal Healing*, by Allen M. Schoen, DVM, and Pam Proctor (Simon & Schuster). This is a marvelously woven text full of tenderness, practicality, insights into the wondrous bond of companionship between animal and man, and finely crafted vignettes that make you want to read more and more. After you read this book you will be better equipped to know when a cherished pet is "ready to let go" and how you can deal with the situation. Available in bookstores.

- *The Complete Herbal Handbook for the Dog and Cat*, by Juliette DeBairacli-Levy (Faber and Faber, London).

- *All You Ever Wanted to Know About Herbs for Pets*, by Gregory L. Tilford and Mary Wulff-Tilford (Bowtie Press, Irvine, CA, 1998; phone: 949-855-8822, ext. 25). This big book is jam-packed with illustrations, photographs, and comprehensive information about the medicinal uses of herbs for pets. If you can accommodate the $50 price tag, the book is a magnificent resource.

- *The Natural Remedy Book for Dogs and Cats*, by Diane Stein (Crossing Press, Freedom, CA, 1994).

- *Are You Poisoning Your Pets?* by Nina Anderson and Howard Peiper (Safe Goods, East Canaan, CT, 1995; phone: 860-824-5301). This is a useful guidebook on how *our* environmentally abusive lifestyles affect the health of pets…and what you can do about it.

- *Super Nutrition for Animals*, by Anderson, Peiper, and Alicia McWatters (Safe Goods, East Canaan, CT, 1996). Nutritional tips for feeding dogs, cats, ferrets, horses, and birds, with many testimonials from animal owners.

- *Raising Healthy Pets: Insights of a Holistic Veterinarian*, by Norman Ralston, DVM (One Peaceful World Press, P.O. Box 10, Leland Rd., Becket, MA 01223; phone: 413-623-2322). At the time of his death in 1999, Dr. Ralston had practiced veterinary medicine for more than half a century. His book includes how macrobiotic principles can be applied to animal health care.

- *Natural Care of Pets*, by Roger DeHaan, DVM, a collection of nearly forty informative articles written by a longtime holistic veterinarian. Subject titles include "Understanding Nutrition," "What Is Acupuncture?" "Animal Chiropractic," "Herbal Medicine and Pet Health," "Skin Problems from A Holistic Viewpoint," "The Missing Ingredient—Food Enzymes," "Stress and Illness—Alleviating Stress," "Making Wise Diet Change Decisions," "Making the Medicine 'Go Down,'" "Puppy Sense—Your New Puppy," and "Home Remedies for Pets." To order this collection send a check or money order for $10.95 to Roger DeHaan, RR1, P.O. Box 47A, Frazee, MN 56544.

- *The Caring Pet Guardian's Guide to Complementary Therapies*, by T. E. Van Cise, DVM, is a fifty-four-page booklet prepared in a lively, concise, question-and-answer form by an experienced California veterinarian. The book covers frequently asked questions about some of the many alternative therapies performed by holistic practitioners, including acupuncture, acuscope therapy, aromatherapy, auricular medicine, color therapy, gold bead implanation, herbal and flower essence therapy, homeopathy, laser and magnetic therapy, Reiki, and Tachyon energy. Available through Dr. Van Cise's clinic in Norco, California. Phone: 909-737-1242.

- *The New Natural Cat*, by Anitra Frazier with Norma Eckroate (Plume, 1990).

- *Cat Care, Naturally*, by Celeste Yarnall. Call 1-888-CEL PETS.

- *Reigning Cats and Dogs* by Pat McKay (Oscar Publications, South Pasadena, CA). Animal nutrition expert McKay has long been a steadfast champion of raw food feeding and supplementation for pets. This book tells you how to feed with fresh, wholesome foods. Call 800-975-7555. If you are interested in the issue of vaccinations, Pat has also put together a book entitled *Natural Immunity*, available at the same number. Web site: http://homel.gte.net/patmckay/index.html.

- *Let's Cook for Our Cat*, by Edmund R. Dorosz, DVM. This book is an excellent primer on all you need to know about feeding your animals. Full of information, including how an animal's digestive tract works, how to tell if your animal is getting a good diet, and how to feed young, old, and overweight animals. Many recipes and solid, practical advice from a veterinarian written in a clear, easy-to-understand style. Available through Our Pets, P.O. Box 2094, Fort MacLeod, Alberta, Canada, T0L 0Z0. Web site: http://www.ourpets.com.

- *It's for the Animals Cook Book*, by Helen McKinnon. This potpourri of recipes, basic holistic information, and directory of resources is available by calling 1-908-537-4144. Web site: http://members.aol.com/ifta2.

Index